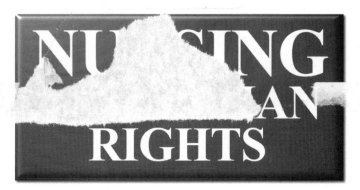

For Butterworth Heinemann:

Commissioning Editor: Susan Young
Development Editor: Catherine Jackson
Project Manager: Ailsa Laing/Temple DPS
Design: George Ajayi

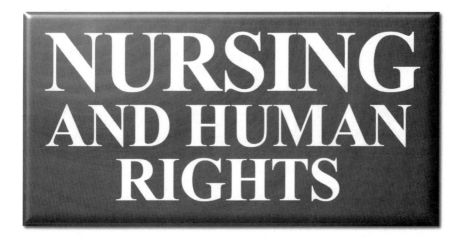

NURSING AND HUMAN RIGHTS

Jean McHale LLB, MPhil

Professor of Law, Faculty of Law, University of Leicester, UK

Ann Gallagher RGN, RMN, BA (Hons), MA, PGCEA

Lecturer in Mental Health, School of Health and Social Welfare,
The Open University, UK

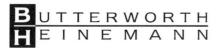

BUTTERWORTH
HEINEMANN

Edinburgh London New York Oxford Philadelphia St Louis Sydney Toronto 2003

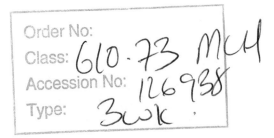
BUTTERWORTH-HEINEMANN
An imprint of Elsevier Limited

First published 2003
    Reprinted 2004

ISBN 0 7506 5292 6

British Library Cataloguing in Publication Data
A catalogue record for this book is available from the British Library

Library of Congress Cataloging in Publication Data
A catalog record for this book is available from the Library of Congress

Note
Medical knowledge is constantly changing. Stantard safety precautions must be followed, but as new research and clinical experience broaden our knowledge, changes in treatment and drug therapy may become necessary or appropriate. Readers are advised to check the most current product information provided by the manufacturer of each drug to be administered to verify the recommended dose, the method and duration of administration, and contraindications. It is the responsibility of the practitioner, relying on experience and knowledge of the patient, to determine dosages and the best treatment for each individual patient. Neither the Publisher nor the authors assumes any liability for any injury and/or damage to persons or property arising from this publication.

 your source for books,
journals and multimedia
in the health sciences
www.elsevierhealth.com

The
publisher's
policy is to use
**paper manufactured
from sustainable forests**

Printed in China
B/02

Contents

Acknowledgements

This book would not have been written without the kindness and encouragement of many people. We would like to thank Mary Seager who initially suggested that we write this text and the rest of the production team at Elsevier Science for their kind assistance – in particular Susan Young and Catherine Jackson – and Jane Bowler at Temple Design.

Several people kindly read through chapters and their thoughts and help are gratefully acknowledged, although of course all errors that remain are ours alone. We would like to thank Anne Arber, Andrew Edgar, Susanne Gibson, Susan Heatley, Maggie Mallik, Chris Middleton and Rena Papadopoulos. Others who provided pointers/advice/support and discussed issues with us, and to whom we are also very grateful, are Bart Cusveller, Theresa Drought, Mary McCann, Claire O'Tuathail and of course Tim Owen for his resolution of all computer emergencies!

Last but by no means least, our families for their help and their patience through the writing process.

Table of cases

ECHR Cases

Statutes and Statutory Instruments

Chapter 1

Human rights and nursing

Introduction

'The Act gives every citizen a clear statement of rights and responsibilities. And it requires all of us in public service to respect human rights in everything we do.' Prime Minister, Tony Blair (Home Office 1999)

In 2002 Diane Pretty sought the assistance of the English courts and the European Convention of Human Rights to assert her ' right to die'. In the same year Diane Blood succeeded in her attempt to get her dead husband's name on the birth certificates of their children who were conceived posthumously using human rights arguments. One year earlier, patients succeeded in obtaining revisions to the powers of mental health tribunals under the Mental Health Act 1983 on the basis of Article 5(3) of the European Court of Human Rights. These are just a few notable examples of the impact of the Human Rights Act 1998 in health care.

The language of rights has long informed the debate surrounding the provision of health care in this country and elsewhere. However, it was the enactment of the Human Rights Act 1998 which forced the recognition of rights onto centre stage and into the public arena. While English citizens already had the right to petition the European Court of Human Rights in Strasbourg, the process was time consuming. Applicants also had to first exhaust the remedies available in the English courts. Moreover, even if the applicant won an action in practice, there was no obligation on the UK government to implement the recommendations, although media pressure might result in consequent changes. While there was a lively debate over many years as to whether a Bill of Rights should be introduced the legislature was resistant to change. Prior to taking office, the Labour Party published 'Bringing Rights Home' (Straw & Boateng 1996), which signalled a different approach. In 1997 the new Labour Government introduced the Human Rights Bill (HMSO 1997) leading to its ultimate enactment in 1998.

Nurses and nursing bodies have long been concerned with ethical practice. The emphasis has, traditionally, been on virtues and duties or obligations rather than rights. The implementation of the Human Rights Act 1998 urges a reconsideration of professional ethics and the role of rights. While much rhetoric surrounded the implementation of the Human Rights Act, the real impact of the Act on nursing practice remains uncertain and will continue to evolve as challenges come through the courts. This book begins to explore some of these issues. In this first chapter we consider: what is meant by 'human rights'; the relationship between rights and health care; the background to and workings of the Human Rights Act 1998; the implications for nurses and nursing of a human rights approach; and the challenges and potential of a rights discourse in health care.

Human rights – from the parochial to the global?

A great deal is claimed on the basis of rights – the right to life, to be free from torture, to free speech, to remain silent, to health, to work, to education, to hunt and so on. Appeals are also made to rights on the basis of belonging to a sub-section of humanity, for example, to women's rights, gay rights, children's rights, to the rights of older people, the mentally ill and to the rights of those who belong to minority groups. Rights are also claimed for animals. The concern of this book is with rights which are bestowed on people simply because they are human – rights which are universal, which treat individuals as equals, which mainly concern the relationship between the individual and the state and which are underpinned by a belief in human dignity. 'Human rights' have a long and distinguished history but their existence also reminds us of human potential for cruelty and as, Glover (1999) puts it, 'man-made horrors'. He says:

'To talk of the twentieth-century atrocities is in one way misleading. It is a myth that barbarism is unique to the twentieth century: the whole of human history includes wars, massacres, and every kind of torture and cruelty: there are grounds for thinking that over much of the world the changes of the last hundred years or so have been towards a psychological climate more humane than at any previous time. But it is still right that much of twentieth-century history has been a very unpleasant surprise. Technology has made a difference. The decisions of a few people can mean horror and death for hundreds of thousands, even millions of other people.' (ibid p.3)

Human rights declarations might be viewed as both a response to, and a means to reduce, if not to eliminate, the possibility of future atrocities. The history of human rights, however, stretches beyond the twentieth century. Three generations, phases or waves of rights have been identified. The French jurist, Vasak, described these as: *liberté; égalité;* and *fraternité* (Austin 2001 p.185). The first wave is described then as the 'libertarian wave', which emerged from the Enlightenment period, a period when there was discussion of the 'natural rights of man' and challenges to religious suppression. This phase was the background to the French and American uprisings in the eighteenth century and resulted in the American Bill of Rights and the French Declaration of the Rights of Man. This first period of human rights was concerned with liberty or civil and political rights.

The second phase or wave of rights was a response to the atrocities of the Second World War and is described as the current era of human rights. While the protection of individual freedoms was still evident in declarations and treaties, the acknowledgement that states and individuals had participated in these atrocities made the inclusion of other values necessary. Values such as dignity, equality and community were central to this second phase or wave. There was a requirement that governments take positive action to secure rights and not just to abstain from interference in the lives of individuals. These rights are described as social and economic as well as civil and political. Klug (2000) points out:

'No issue was considered more relevant to this approach than discrimination, and racial discrimination in particular. The Nazi Holocaust against the Jews and other minorities influenced every aspect of the deliberations of the drafters of the 1948 Universal Declaration of Human Rights, leading to a new emphasis of the value of equality. This approach was to change the way that human rights defenders viewed the principle of liberty. Once people are told they cannot be free to choose who to let their house to or who to hire and fire if their choice is based on racial or sexual discrimination, for example, then freedom takes on a new and more complex meaning.' (ibid p.11)

The third phase or wave of rights has been defined variously. Vasak (cited by Austin 2001 p.185) defined the third phase as *fraternité* or solidarity which was viewed as a response to market forces under globalisation. Solidarity rights or global solidarity rights are said to propose that 'there should be a global reallocation of resources' so that poorer countries have the means to build the necessary institutions to protect human rights (Wilkinson & Caulfield 2000 p.3). Solidarity rights are also taken to include the right to a clean environment and to peace. Klug (2000) has a different interpretation of the third wave of rights. She says:

'While there is still the same recognition of the values of liberty and community as in the second wave, there is now a growing emphasis on participation and mutuality... More definitively as at the dawn of the second wave, it is now established that states are not the only, or always the main, abusers of power. As significantly, there is a new emphasis on seeking change through trade agreements, education and persuasion as well as through litigation. A cross-cultural dialogue on human rights is developing which involves a far wider set of participants than the jurists and standard-setters who dominated the second wave. In essence this fledgling third wave does not so much involve a change in the characterisation of rights as an evolution in the place of rights in society.' (ibid p.12)

Later, Klug writes of the increased participation of people in rights debates and links the value of mutuality with the third wave of rights:

'Because of this participation – and because rights are increasingly presented as more than claims against governments but also as a set of obligations that individuals owe to each other – a new value of mutuality can be said to characterise an emerging third wave of rights.' (ibid p.196)

Discussing the third wave of rights in terms of mutuality responds to a major criticism levied at a rights approach – that is, that a rights approach pays little or no attention to corresponding obligations or duties.

Thus far, we have said something about the background to the evolution of human rights. Short of an extensive empirical study, it is not possible to know for sure how human rights are viewed by the general population or, indeed, by nurses and other health care professionals. It has been suggested that there is a view of human rights as concerning other countries and not to do with everyday local issues. Klug again writes:

'Ask most people in this country and they would probably say that human rights are something that foreigners lack. They are about torture, disappearances, arbitrary detentions, unfair trials and so forth; outrages which are not within the personal experiences of the vast majority of people in a country like the UK... In other words, they seem to be saying, human rights have got nothing to do with what goes on in the courts or police stations of the UK, let alone in classrooms or residential homes. Yet the jurisprudence, or case law, of the European Court of Human Rights is entirely consistent with a growing trend in international human rights thinking that human rights principles can be meaningfully applied to situations that face us all in our everyday lives.' (Klug 2000 p.5)

What the discussion surrounding the Human Rights Act 1998, and the cases which are fought on the basis of it, should emphasise is that human rights are very much related to our everyday lives – as citizens, professionals and patients. This does not mean, however, that we become morally myopic focusing only on local issues. Human rights are for all humans – wherever and however they live. An awareness of this and a need to consider the implications of taking rights seriously is made all the more pressing by the forces of globalisation. As Leaning (2001) writes:

'Globalisation, by providing a commercial and technological engine for the movement of people, capital, and information, has accelerated and complicated issues of social proximity. More than ever the world, in all its diversity and pain, is at our doorsteps.' (ibid pp.1435-6)

The historical development of rights has then, it can be argued, moved from an emphasis on individual freedoms and liberty to an emphasis on equality and non-discrimination to an era of rights which emphasises mutuality and participation. This is a view of human rights which includes human obligations and duties. These three waves can be seen to co-exist in contemporary rights documents. Since the inception of human rights many treaties and declarations have been developed and ratified. A good number of these make reference to the right to health.

Rights and health care

It has been suggested that 'modern concepts of both health and human rights are complex and steadily evolving' (Mann et al 1999, Chapter 1). We have outlined three phases or waves of rights and it seems plausible that there will be other phases and other rights identified in the future which are in keeping with societal and global changes. In this section, we will consider views of health and discuss interpretations of the 'right to health'.

Three relationships have been suggested between health and human rights (Mann et al 1999, Chapter 1). First, health policies and practices have the potential to impact, positively or negatively, on human rights. Mental health policy, for example, permits the exercise of government power both to promote the welfare of the individual, the family and society and also to deprive individuals of their right to liberty, privacy and property. Policies regarding resource allocation may also disadvantage some groups (for example, older people) resulting in a deterioration of health. Second, rights violations such as torture, abuse, neglect and violations of privacy can have a detrimental impact on health, particularly mental health. Finally, the positive promotion of human rights and health are 'inextricably linked' in that they are both concerned with the well-being of human beings. It has been pointed out that:

'health and human rights are both powerful approaches to defining and advancing human well-being.' (ibid p.7)

There is no consensus as to what health involves but two broad views are apparent in the literature – a medical view and a social view. A medical or 'engineering' model of health conceives of the body as a machine and focuses on disease rather than wellbeing or health promotion (Montgomery 1992). A broader view is evident in the World Health Organisation definition of health:

'a state of complete physical, mental and social well-being and not merely the absence of disease and infirmity.' (WHO 1948)

This is sometimes referred to as a social or holistic model of health and defines health as an ideal state. This definition has been criticised for its idealism. On this account few, if any of us, would qualify as healthy. This broad definition can be contrasted with the medical or engineering view – whereas a medical curative model will require that professional activities are concentrated on acute services and treatments, a social model of health will involve professionals in health promotion and family health services. With a broader social view of health, attention also needs to be paid to other sectors which make a significant contribution to health but which are not generally thought of as 'health care'.

Where a right to health or health care is claimed, it is clearly significant which view of health is proposed. Montgomery (1992) indicates that a broader perspective may be preferable. He suggests that those 'rights which are required by the narrower model will almost certainly be also required by the broader one'. The broader model links to other factors such as poor housing, poverty, education, the environment and socio-economic class. He suggests that such a model would encompass four broad categories:

- protection from disease and accident, including public health measures and also measures contained in the criminal law penalising violence
- protection from adverse environmental factors
- the promotion of a healthy environment, and
- the provision of health care services.

However, a broad definition of 'health' may in practice lead to considerable problems regarding enforcement. As Gostin and Lazzarini (1997) commented:

'A right to health that is too broadly defined lacks clear content and is less likely to have any meaningful impact.'

They propose an alternative approach; that the right to health may be regarded as:

'[t]he duty of the state within the limits of its available resources to ensure the conditions necessary for the health of individuals and populations.'

Gostin and Lazzarini note that many factors which impact upon the individual's state of health are beyond governmental control, such as genetics, behaviour, over-population and climate. Nonetheless, as they argue, it is the State which possesses the power to ensure conditions under which people are healthy through such things as the provision of decent sanitation, hygiene, clean air, clean water, nutrition, clothing, housing and medical services. They suggest that the State would have a responsibility within the limits of available resources to intervene to prevent or reduce serious threats to the health of individuals and populations. Nonetheless, as they recognise, a disadvantage with such an approach is that it does not ensure a minimal standard of health. It also sanctions differential responses to threats to health based upon available economic resources.

It seems clear that arguing for a right to health defined as the ideal state of the World Health Organisation is not achievable and attempts to strive towards this would quickly exhaust state resources. A medical view of the right to health is also inadequate as medical treatment is not necessarily the main contributor to health. Gostin and Lazzarini's arguments for the conditions necessary for health, based on state resources, is also question-begging – how is health defined? If defined broadly, then some might claim a right to fertility treatment or cosmetic surgery. Also, how is it to be decided how much of state resources are to be devoted to health? Britain currently devotes much less of its Gross National Product (GNP) to health than most other Western countries. Defining health and drawing conclusions about what the right to health involves is then no easy matter. It is important to distinguish between the 'right to health' which includes the socio-economic factors which contribute to healthy living and 'access rights', the right to access health care.

In writing of the 'right to health' Austin (2001) points out:

'Taken literally, a right to health makes little sense: no government can guarantee the health of a citizen. The right to health, however, is actually shorthand in rights discourse for the more complex terminology of international treatises and documents.' (ibid p.185)

So how does the right to health and/or health care appear in international treatises and declarations?

In 1946, through the adoption of the World Health Organisation's Constitution, countries accepted the fundamental right to 'the enjoyment of the highest attainable standard of health'. Article 25 of the Universal Declaration of Human Rights (UDHR 1948) stated:

'Everyone has the right to a standard of living adequate for the health and well being of himself and his family including food, clothing, housing and medical care and the right to security in the event of unemployment, sickness, disability, widowhood, old age or other lack of livelihood in circumstances beyond his control.'

Other Articles in the UDHR also have relevance to the right to health. Article 3 provides that 'Everyone has a right to life' and Article 5 that 'No one shall be subject to torture or to inhuman or degrading treatment or punishment'.

Other international statements which make direct or indirect reference to health rights or their provisions may be applicable in relation to arguments to the effect that patients should be accorded a particular standard of health care.

The International Covenant on Civil and Political Rights (ICCPR 1976) provides that there is an 'inherent right to life protected by law' (Article 1), and that 'All persons deprived of their liberty shall be treated with respect for the inherent dignity of the human person' (Article 10).

Such prohibition on torture, inhuman and degrading treatment is a fundamental non-derogable right. This may be applicable in the health context; for example, restrictions/limitations placed upon persons with HIV/AIDS. It may also be applicable in a situation in which a severely incapacitated person is denied access to euthanasia. Other traditional civil and political rights, which may be applicable in the health context, include the right to privacy and rights to freedom of conscience/religion.

The International Covenant on Economic, Social and Cultural Rights (ICESCR 1976) provides that:

'The States parties to the present Covenant recognise the right of everyone to the enjoyment of the highest ascertainable standard of physical and mental health.' (Article 12(1))

This includes:

'The provision for the reduction of the still birth rate and of infant mortality and for healthy development of the child;

The improvement of all aspects of environmental and industrial hygiene;

The prevention, treatment and control of epidemic, endemic, occupational and other diseases;

The creation of conditions which would assure to all medical service and medical attention in the event of sickness.'

The Covenant provides that:

'[the] State may subject such rights only to such limitations as are determined by law only in so far as this may be compatible with the nature of these rights and solely for the purpose of promoting the general welfare in a democratic society.' (Article 4)

The UDHR, the ICCPR and the ICESPR together with the First and Second Protocols to the ICCPR comprise the International Bill of Human Rights.

Certain other declarations recognise rights in relation to treatment. The Convention for the Protection of Human Rights and Dignity of the Human Being with Regard to the Application of Biology and Medicine (1997), which has not yet been signed by the United Kingdom, sets out a series of patient rights. It states in Article 1 that the purpose and object is safeguarding the dignity and identity of all human beings and respecting their integrity and other fundamental rights and freedoms. Provisions make reference to such matters as consent (Articles 5-9), private life and the right to information (Article 12), controls on genetics and prohibition of discrimination (Articles 11-13), research (Articles 15-18) and removal of organs and tissues from living donors for transplantation purposes (Articles 21-22) (see further Zilgavis (2002)).

The Convention on the Rights of the Child (UN 1989) (one of the international documents which has received the largest number of ratifications – over 190) provides, in Articles 5 and 12, a duty to respect the evolving capacities of the child and to give the child's views due weight according to their age and maturity. Explicit provisions referring to consent with regards to experimentation are not included in the Convention.

The European Union Charter on Fundamental Freedoms, which is not yet a legally binding document, makes reference to many of the traditional civil and political rights in addition to certain rights of specific relevance in the health context. For example, this provides under the heading 'Dignity' in Chapter 1 the following provisions:

'Article 3(2)

In the fields of medicine/biology the following must be respected:

1. Free informed consent of the person concerned according to the procedures laid down by law.

2. The prohibition on eugenic practices, in particular those aiming at the selection of persons.

3. The prohibition on making the human body and its parts as such a source of financial gain.

4. The prohibition of the reproductive cloning of human beings.'

Under the heading 'Freedoms' reference is made to the rights of liberty and security of the person, the right to marry, freedom of conscience, freedom of expression and the right to privacy. Under Chapter 4, 'Solidarity', which contains many of the 'social' rights, reference is made to a 'right to health care'. This is likely to prove an important statement should this become a binding part of EU law in formulating health care law across the European Union.

More specific and recent comment on the right to health is contained in the UN general comment of Article 12 of the ICESCR (E.C.12.2000/4, CESCR, general comment 14). Here health is defined as a 'fundamental right indispensable for the exercise of other human rights'. In elaborating on 'the normative content' of the right to health it is pointed out that:

'8. The right to health is not to be understood as a right to be healthy. The right to health includes both freedoms and entitlements. The freedoms include the right to control one's health and body, including sexual and reproductive freedom, and the right to be free from interference, such as the right to be free from torture, non-consensual medical treatment and experimentation. By contrast, the entitlements include the right to a system of health protection which provides equality of opportunity for people to enjoy the highest attainable level of health.

9. The notion of 'the highest attainable standard of health' in Article 12.1 takes into account both the individual's biological and socio-economic preconditions and a State's available resources. There are a

number of aspects which cannot be addressed solely within the relationship between States and individuals; in particular, good health cannot be ensured by a State, nor can States provide protection against every possible cause of ill health. Thus, genetic factors, individual susceptibility to ill health and the adoption of unhealthy or risky lifestyles may play an important role with respect to an individual's health. Consequently, the right to health must be understood as a right to the enjoyment of a variety of facilities, goods, services and conditions necessary for the realisation of the highest attainable standard of health.'

Four elements of the right to health are identified: availability (functioning public health and health care facilities, goods, services and programmes including safe water and sanitation); accessibility (facilities, goods and services have to be available to all without discrimination); acceptability (facilities, goods and services must be respectful of medical ethics and culturally appropriate); and quality (facilities, goods and services must be scientifically and medically appropriate and of good quality) (http:// www..../E.C.12.2000.4,+CESCR+General+comment+14.En?OpenDocumen).

It is further acknowledged that the right to health is:

'closely related to and dependent on the realisation of other human rights, as contained in the International Bill of Rights, including the rights to food, housing, work, education, human dignity, life, non-discrimination, equality, the prohibition against torture, privacy, access to information, and the freedom of association, assembly and movement. These and other rights and freedoms address integral components of the right to health.' (ibid Section 3)

Until 2000 these various international and European provisions had only limited impact in UK law. There was no one single comprehensive Bill of Human Rights (although there is one earlier Bill of Rights enacted in 1688; this was very limited in its content, though reference was made to the prohibition on cruel and unusual punishment in decided cases). The most important statement which had an impact upon English law and policy was the European Convention of Human Rights.

The European Convention of Human Rights and European Court of Human Rights

The Convention for the Protection of Human Rights and Fundamental Freedoms, drawn up by the Council of Europe, was produced in 1950 (Overs & White 2002). This was an attempt to begin the enforcement in Europe of some of those rights contained in the Universal Declaration of Human Rights which had been signed in 1948. The enforcement of those rights was undertaken by the European Commission of Human Rights established in 1954, the European Court of Human Rights (established in 1959) and the

Committee of the Ministers of the Council of Europe (this was the Foreign Affairs ministers of member states and their representatives). If a state accepted what was known as the 'right of individual petition' then individual applicants could bring an action against states who had contracted to be part of the ECHR claiming that ECHR rights had been infringed. Initially these cases were examined by the Commission. Where they were held to be admissible the Commission would draw up a report and would submit this to the Committee of Ministers. In addition, in a situation in which a state had also contracted to be part of the jurisdiction of the Court, the Commission or any contracting state could refer the case to the European Court of Human Rights. An individual citizen, however, could not bring an action.

The problem with proceedings before the Commission and Court was the case load, which steadily increased and which ultimately led to long delays in dealing with applications. This led to calls for reform of the structure. In May 1994, Protocol 11 to the European Convention on Human Rights 'Restructuring the Control Machinery' was opened for signature. This document had to be ratified by all signing states which was ultimately completed in October 1997. It simplified the system – the role of the Committee of Ministers was abolished and instead one single full-time court was created, which was a much larger body than its predecessor. Another important difference was that a member state or an individual who alleged that their rights had been infringed could bring an action before the Court. An individual may bring proceedings themselves although legal representation is encouraged and there is a legal aid system available established by the Council of Europe where applicants have insufficient means.

The Human Rights Act 1998 – background and workings

While UK citizens could petition the ECHR the procedure was time consuming and, moreover, the rulings of the European Court of Human Rights were not binding upon the UK government who could, in theory at least, choose to disregard its ruling. While the English courts had shown some receptivity to ECHR principles prior to the enactment of the 1998 Act, the Convention was not binding in UK courts (*R v Secretary of State for the Home Department ex parte Brind* [1991] AC 696). The Human Rights Act 1998 now provides a mechanism by which health care rights can be challenged in the English courts. The effect of the Act is to direct English courts to those rights set out in the European Convention of Human Rights (1950). The 1998 Act allows for the Convention rights to become operative in the English courts. Interestingly, Section 19 of the Act also provides that where a government minister is introducing legislation into Parliament they must provide a written statement before the second reading regarding the compatibility of the proposed legislation with Convention rights. This provision again emphasises the importance given to the legislation. In addition to drawing attention to the new developments through extensive professional judicial training in relation to the operation of the Act, a Human Rights Unit was established by the Home Office in addition to the creation of a Joint Ministerial/Non-Governmental Rights Task Force.

In the next section, we will outline: the nature of the rights within the HRA 1998; its scope of application; the nature of interpretation; and the significance of the declaration of incompatibility.

Categories of rights

The 1998 Act covers different categories of rights. Not all the rights included in the European Convention of Human Rights itself were enacted. It is important to note that while the rights were included initially in the Convention, decades ago, the Convention is interpreted in the light of contemporary society rather than the relevant mores of the society when the Convention was first drafted.

Certain rights are absolute in nature and cannot be restricted such as Article 2, the right to life. Another such right is Article 3, the prohibition upon torture and inhuman and degrading treatment. Illustrations of cases in which Article 2 applications are likely concern decision making at the end of life, particularly regarding assisted suicide (such as the Diane Pretty case) and decisions to withdraw treatment and also regarding abortion. The potential application of Article 3 is also broad. The European Court of Human Rights has defined 'torture' as being 'deliberate inhuman treatment causing very serious and cruel suffering'. Inhuman treatment relates to 'at least such treatment as deliberately causes severe suffering, mental or physical which in the particular situation is unjustifiable'. Moreover, the European Court of Human Rights has gone on to state that 'treatment of an individual may be said to be degrading if it grossly humiliates him before others or drives him to act against his own will or conscience' (*Ireland v UK* (1979-1980) 2 EHRR 25).

Horton has suggested that:

> 'Doctors seeing patients who come from the most vulnerable groups in society – the old, children, the poor, those in prison – may now have an explicit obligation to draw attention to instances when the rights of these individuals are ignored or neglected. Those parts of the National Health Service and social services that bring patients perilously close to conditions that are degrading are ripe for challenge.' (Horton 2000)

While the courts may be receptive to the application of rights analysis regarding treatment decisions, when issues of resource allocation arise the use of such statements is more problematic. The courts have, in many instances, been unwilling to uphold claims based upon access to particular forms of health care (see Chapter 6 regarding rights and resources).

A second category of rights is known as 'limited rights' such as Article 5 – liberty and security of the person. Here the right is established but the Article contains a long series of legitimate exceptions, for example, including in paragraph (e) the lawful detention of persons for the prevention of the spreading of infectious diseases, of persons of unsound mind, alcoholics or drug addicts or vagrants. There has already been considerable use of this provision in the context of those persons with mental illness (see for example *R v Camden and Islington HA ex parte K* The Times 15th March 2001).

Thirdly, there is a group known as 'qualified rights'. This is the group of Articles between Articles 8 (the right to privacy), Article 9 (freedom of conscience and religion) and Article 10 (freedom of expression). They may be qualified where the interference is in accordance with the law or where it is necessary in a democratic society in the interests of national security/public safety, prevention of crime/disorder or the protection of health or morals. It is important to note that in considering whether the limitations apply 'there must be a reasonable relationship of proportionality between the means employed and the legitimate objectives pursued by the collective limitations' (*Fayed v UK* (1994) 18 EHRR 393 at 432).

These 'qualified' rights are applicable in the health care context in a range of situations. Article 8 has considerable implications in relation to decisions of consent and refusal of treatment and confidentiality of health care information. In conjunction with Article 12 (the right to marry and found a family), Article 8 has application in relation to access to infertility treatment. Article 9 is particularly applicable in relation to the right of health care professionals to claim that they can opt out of certain procedures on the basis of conscientious objection. Equally, it applies to those patients, whether adults or children, who refuse clinical procedures on the basis that these procedures infringe tenets of their faith.

Bringing an action under the Human Rights Act 1998

Section 6 provides that the Human Rights Act 1998 applies to public authorities which include NHS bodies. There has been considerable debate as to whether it also has a horizontal effect and thus extends to activities between private individuals (Buxton 2000; Wade 2000; Hunt 1998). An action under the Human Rights Act 1998 may be brought by someone who is a victim of an unlawful act by a public authority (Sections 7(1) and 7(3)). Section 7 applies to those who are directly affected. The extent and application of this provision has been the subject of critical comment (see, for example, Whitty, Murphy & Livingstone 2001 at page 31). It is not as broad as the tests used in judicial review enabling a person to bring proceedings where they have 'sufficient interest' to bring such an action. The test for bringing proceedings before the ECHR itself is also broader. It has been suggested that one approach to the limitations posed by the test as presently structured would be for Non-Governmental Organisations to continue funding litigation through the identification of an individual as a suitable 'victim'. However, there is a further problem with recognition of a broad test, as Whitty, Murphy and Livingstone comment, namely the role of private groups who are challenging the actions of private individuals, for example, the anti-abortion group. They argue for a context-sensitive application of the rules of standing which they suggest would 'offer one potential safeguard against pressure-group litigation which has as its aim the deliberate undermining of other core rights and values presented by the HRA (such as privacy and equality rights of women, lesbians or gays) (Whitty, Murphy & Livingstone 2002 at page 33).

There is a new right of action provided against a public body acting in a public capacity such as an NHS body which acts in a manner which is incompatible with a right under the ECHR (Sections 6(1) and 7(1) Human Rights Act 1998). An action may be possible for judicial review, for breach of statutory duty or as a defence in an action against a public body. Damages may be awarded in a situation in which in all the circumstances of the case it is necessary to award 'just satisfaction' to the victim (Section 8(2)). It should be noted that the remedies available are only as extensive as the existing powers of the court.

The declaration of incompatibility

Where legislation is inconsistent the court may disapply (in effect to set aside) subordinate legislation such as statutory instruments. This applies as long as the legislation does not prevent this. What the court cannot do is strike down primary legislation and in effect act as a 'Supreme Court' in that situation. The word of Parliament, as expressed through statute, ultimately prevails. Nonetheless the Act provides certain courts such as the House of Lords, High Court and county courts with the power to make what is called a 'declaration of incompatibility' (Section 4(2)). As a consequence of such a declaration of incompatibility a government minister may make a 'remedial order' in relation to a particular piece of legislation, although this is not automatic and is not binding, rather it is discretionary (Section 10). In the debates on the Act Jack Straw gave an example of the Abortion Act as being the type of situation in which a remedial order would be unlikely (317 HC 1301 (21 Oct 1998)). The first illustration of such a declaration concerning health care matters was that of *R (H) v Mental Health Review Tribunal North and East London Region and another* ([2001] HRLR 36). H was detained in a secure hospital, subject to restrictions under Sections 37 and 41 of the Mental Health Act 1983 after having been convicted of manslaughter. He applied to a tribunal to be discharged. The tribunal refused to discharge him and his application for judicial review of the decision of the tribunal was refused. The Court of Appeal held that Sections 72 and 73 contravened Article 5 of the European Convention of Human Rights. Lord Phillips MR stated that the provisions were in conflict with Article 5(4) because the burden of proof rests on the patient to show that he no longer suffered from a mental disorder which warranted his continued detention. The burden of proof and the test for discharge could not be separated. The Mental Health Act 1983, in failing to require a tribunal to discharge a patient, constituted unlawful detention and this constituted an infringement of an individual's right to liberty. Nonetheless, although the declaration has been made, the statutory provisions themselves were still initially applicable because the Act did not allow the courts to strike down primary legislation. However, subsequently, regulations have been issued to amend the provisions of the Mental Health Act 1983 accordingly.

How the courts interpret the ECHR

First, where an English court is determining a matter 'in connection with' a right under the Convention then it must, as far as is applicable, take account of case law from the European Court of Human Rights (Human Rights Act 1998 Section 2). In *R (Alconbury Developments Ltd) v Environment Secretary* ([2001] 2 WLR 1389) Lord Slynn held that 'In the absence of some special circumstances it seems to me that the court should follow any clear and constant jurisprudence of the European Court of Human Rights'. The type of situation which may fall under the 'special circumstances' category was highlighted by Lord Hoffman. He commented that:

'The House is not bound by the decisions of the European Court and if I thought... they compelled a conclusion fundamentally at odds with the distribution of powers under the British Constitution, I would have considerable doubts as to whether they should be followed.'

Similarly in *Aston Cantlow Parochial Church Council v Wallbank* [2001] 3 All ER 393 the Court of Appeal held that their task was:

'In the light of Section 2(1) of the Human Rights Act 1998 it is to draw out the broad principles which animate the Convention.'

Second, all primary and secondary legislation must be 'read and given effect to in a way which is compatible with Convention rights' (Section 3). But what does that mean; exactly how far can the courts go in such a situation? In *R v A (No 2)* [2001] 2 WLR 1546 Lord Steyn emphasised that a declaration of incompatibility should be seen as a measure of 'last resort' and that if necessary the words of a statute could be 'linguistically strained' to read them consistently with the ECHR. This could mean, for example, that the court when interpreting a statute could imply provisions. Further consideration was given to the use of Section 3 in *R v Lambert* ([2001] 3 WLR 206). Here Lord Hope indicated that Section 3 would not be applicable if to do so would be to expressly contradict the express provisions of the statute. The court would have to take great care when construing the provision of the statute to ensure that this was compatible. One approach was that of expressing the words in a different way or through reading in other words – although this could not be undertaken as amendment of the statute.

In *Poplar Housing and Regeneration Community Association Ltd v Donoghue* [2001] EWCA Civ 595 Lord Woolf took the view that Section 3 did not allow courts to legislate but to interpret. He indicated that if it was the case that it would be necessary to 'radically alter' the effect of a statute this would go beyond interpretation. Thus his Lordship was of the view that the Section could not be used where it would have the effect that it would 'defeat Parliament's original objective'.

Third, there is the application of the principle of proportionality. In Articles such as 8, 9 and 10 these are qualified by the fact that measures may be taken where these are necessary 'in the interests of a democratic society' and where this is the case these measures must themselves respond to what is a pressing social need. As Lewis (2001) comments: 'Thus the ECHR seeks to strike the desperately difficult balance between individual human rights and the interests of society at large'.

Fourthly, when cases are being interpreted at ECHR level these are subject to a 'margin of appreciation' which is given by the ECHR to member states. States are given some discretion in the interpretation and application of Convention provisions. However at individual state level it may not be applicable. In *R v DPP ex parte Kebeline* [1999] 3 WLR 972 Lord Hope stated that this doctrine 'was not available to the national courts when they are considering Convention issues arising within their own countries'; it is only relevant in terms of external ECHR scrutiny of particular countries.

Nursing and human rights

The International Council of Nursing position statement regarding nursing and human rights (See http://www.icn.ch/pshumrights.htm; reprinted in Nursing Ethics 2001 8(3) pp. 272-3) is as follows:

> 'Human rights in health care involve both recipients and providers. The International Council of Nurses (ICN) views health care as a right of all individuals, regardless of financial, political, geographic, racial or religious considerations. This right includes the right to choose or decline care, including the right to accept or refuse treatment or nourishment; informed consent; confidentiality, and dignity, including the right to die with dignity.'

As part of professional accountability, the ICN points out, nurses have an obligation to safeguard human rights in relation to health and national nurses' organisations have a responsibility to take part in the development of legislation relating to patients' rights. The ICN also acknowledges nurses' rights as follows:

> 'Nurses have the right to practice in accordance with the nursing legislation of the country in which they work and to adopt the ICN Code for Nurses or their own national ethical code. Nurses also have a right to practice in an environment that provides personal safety, freedom from abuse, violence, threats or intimidation.'

The ICN points to the everyday nature of human rights and to the need for vigilance regarding the ways new technology and research can violate human rights. The Council also points to the need for nurses to understand human rights declarations; to raise awareness of the 'vital link' between health and human rights; to include human rights and ethics education on the professional curriculum; and the need to assume a more political role in lobbying for equitable and universal access to health care.

It has been pointed out that 'ethics has never been a fad in nursing; it has been the very foundation of nursing practice since the inception of modern nursing in the United States in the late 1870s' (Fowler in Davis et al 1997). This also applies to nursing in Britain. Traditionally, the focus of ethics in nursing was on the moral character traits of the nurse (a virtue approach). It should be said that there has been a revival of virtue ethics in recent years and some discussion of virtues in relation to nursing (Lutzen & Barbosa da Silva 1996, Sellman 1997). This was then replaced by a focus on duty or obligation which is evident in professional codes. The recent NMC Code of Professional Conduct (2002) continues to focus on nurses' duties and obligations, but does highlight patients'/clients' rights to receive information (Section 3.1) and to decide whether or not to undergo any health care intervention (Section 3.2). With the incorporation of the HRA 1998 into British law, it is likely that nurses will become much more aware of the implications of rights in health care.

The relationship between nurses and human rights can be characterised variously. Nurses are involved in the promotion of human rights. In addition to everyday examples of nursing actions which respect the human rights of patients (via advocacy, for example), some nurses have endured great personal hardship in efforts to promote the human rights of others (see Citations for Human Rights and Nursing awards in Nursing Ethics (2001 8(3)).

Nurses, sadly, have also been involved in human rights abuses. The work of Hilde Steppe (Chapter 1 in Rafferty et al 1997), for example, details the role of nurses in the Holocaust. Cases of professional misconduct (for example, patient abuse or neglect) which come before the Professional Conduct Committee of the NMC may also constitute violations of human rights.

Nurses have also suffered from human rights abuses. The apartheid system in South Africa, for example, made it very difficult, if not impossible, for non-white nurses to progress in the profession.

Nurses have an important role to play in promoting human rights. This does not require that other approaches to professional ethics are thrown out. Codes should, and can, be supportive of human rights in that they outline the correlative duties or obligations to nurses. A human rights approach requires a broader view – nurses also have rights. Also, a human rights approach entails a less myopic approach – a looking outwards towards more global issues. Human rights is about everyday local concerns but also about the alleviation of suffering and safety of those who migrate here and those in other countries. Education has an important role in promoting human rights in health care.

The prospects for rights in health care – challenges and potential

Klug (2000) has argued that 'the modern idea of human rights has to be understood as a quest for common values in an era of failed ideologies and multiple (including non-existent) faiths'. Nurses work in an increasingly multi-cultural and multi-faith society and need to consider the significance of ethical and legal norms in relation to the needs and values of those who hold different cultural and religious values. Whilst a rights perspective has much to contribute in offering a universal framework for values, it needs to be acknowledged that Articles may be interpreted variously.

A number of specific challenges have been identified in relation to a rights perspective (see, for example, Johnstone 1999, Chapter 4). These include problems of conflicts between rights; reconciling the rights of individuals with the rights and/or needs of others; questions of scope; and in relation to the adequacy of rights as a moral theory.

In health care there may be conflict between, for example, Articles 8 (right to respect for private and family life) and 10 (freedom of expression). This could arise where a professional blows the whistle on poor practice, breaching confidentiality in the process albeit, it might be argued, in the public interest. There is also the potential for conflict between Articles 2 (right to life) and 3 (prohibition of torture, inhuman or degrading treatment) in cases where the patient and/or his or her family wish to continue treatment considered burdensome and futile, on the basis of a right to life. Reconciling the rights of individuals with the rights of others is illustrated throughout the book. Particularly challenging issues arise, for example, in relation to abortion – the rights of the woman may be pitted against the rights of the foetus and/or potential father. In relation to mental health, individuals may be deprived of their liberty to safeguard the lives and well-being of others. In resource allocation, an individual may request an expensive treatment which may lead to fewer resources for others. In relation to the issue of scope, there may be questions about the allocation of rights – to whom/what do they apply? With human rights, it might simply be said that rights apply to humans but might we apply rights to incompetent humans, to the dead, or to body parts and tissue?

Regarding the adequacy of rights as a moral theory, it has been argued that a rights approach is:

> 'not a complete moral theory, but rather (as) a statement of certain minimal and enforceable rules that communities and individuals must observe in their treatment of all persons.' (Beauchamp & Childress 2001 p.361)

It can be argued that whilst human rights is necessary in outlining and reinforcing crucial values such as dignity and autonomy, it is not sufficient. Other ethical approaches are compatible with human rights. Codes of conduct are generally couched in terms of duty or obligation, for example. In which case, duty requirements of the NMC Codes should be compatible with the requirements of the HRA 1998. On a virtue account, it could be argued that professionals need certain moral character traits to be able to adhere to and promote rights adequately. Traits or virtues such as courage, compassion and prudence are particularly relevant here. There is not necessarily any incompatibility between approaches to professional ethics based on rights and those based on obligations or duties. Both approaches also have a legal foundation. Nurses have, for example, a duty of care towards patients and are also required to respect and promote the rights outlined in the HRA 1998.

While the advent of the Human Rights Act was welcomed by many, there were criticisms. Some saw the powers given to the judiciary as too limited in contrast to the Bill of Rights model adopted in other states such as Canada and the USA. Others such as Kentridge (1998) suggested that the ECHR was not necessarily the appropriate model to adopt. Kentridge argued that the Act 'is a mid-century bill of rights designed to accommodate a number of countries with a variety of legal systems and political histories'. Some also note the problems with certain provisions such as Section 3 where the perceived concentration on technical principles of interpretation can be rather seen as unduly limited rather than instead as a new approach giving the courts flexibility (Whitty, Murphy & Livingstone 2001 at page 26).

Some concerns also relate to the role of the judiciary themselves in interpretation of human rights matters. How would the judiciary use the new tools given to it (McGoldrick 2001)? The English judiciary has come under much criticism for its politicisation and the fact that the judiciary were traditionally drawn from a narrow background – white, male, middle-class and Oxbridge educated (Griffiths 1997). It will be interesting to see over the next decade how creatively the judiciary responds to the challenges of the legislation.

Conclusions – where has the Act taken us and where are we going in the future?

The enactment of human rights legislation into English law, in the form of the Human Rights Act 1998, has led to a myriad of cases in which the courts are asked to deal with issues of rights regarding health-related issues. But while the number of cases in which such issues have been raised has been considerable, its impact in practice may be regarded as having been rather more limited. Research on the operation of the first year of the Human Rights Act has indicated that in practice there are only a few cases which have been brought which rely solely on a human rights point (Klug & Starmer 2001). Researchers at the Human Rights Act Research Unit at Kings College London examined 149 cases between October 2nd 2000 and May 24th 2001 where the Act was substantively considered and found that in 85 cases the Act had some effect on the outcome, the reasoning or the procedure. However in only 24 cases was a claim under the Act actually upheld.

Interestingly the research noted that 16 of these cases related to the Section 6 duty noted above. This requires public authorities to act in compliance with the Convention. A further six concerned the requirement to interpret legislation compatibly with the Convention. Two cases led to a declaration of incompatibility.

Many of the cases discussed in this book relate to the period after this research was undertaken. However, as we shall see, while the Act has provided a useful framework for the development of the law in this area it has been far from the radical reforming tool that some might have envisaged from the fanfare surrounding its introduction. Perhaps, though, this is not surprising. For litigators exploring the potential for effective application of human rights challenges in this country may take some time. Radical development of the law in the light of the Human Rights Act may also require a leap of faith on the part of the English judiciary. It also needs to be emphasised that, as noted above, the House of Lords is not a Supreme Court; the Human Rights Act provides tools to change the approach in many areas but it does not enable the judiciary to embark on wholesale legislative reform. But the very existence of a Human Rights Act may have one very positive effect, namely in changing people's attitudes and expectations and introducing a human rights culture (McGoldrick 2001). As Lord Irving the Lord Chancellor commented:

'The objective of the Human Rights Act is to promote a culture of respect for human rights and responsibilities which over time will permeate the whole of our institutions and society.' ('Government to Bring Rights Home' (2000) Press Release, 12 July)

The powerful impact that the very rhetoric of rights can have should not be underestimated.

References

Austin W 2001 Using the human rights paradigm in health ethics: the problems and the possibilities. Nursing Ethics 8(3): 183-195
Beauchamp T, Childress 2001 Principles of biomedical ethics. Oxford University Press, Oxford.
Blair T 1999 Conventional behaviour: questions about the Human Rights Act, an introduction for public authorities. Home Office, London
Buxton R 2000 The Human Rights Act and private law. LQR 48
Davis A J, Aroskar M A, Liaschenko J et al 1997 Ethical dilemmas and nursing practice, 4th edn. Appleton & Lange, Stamford
Glover 1999 Humanity – A moral history of the twentieth century. Jonathan Cape, London
Gostin L, Lazzarini Z 1997 Human rights and public health in the AIDS pandemic. Oxford University Press, Oxford
Griffiths J 1997 Politics of the judiciary. Fontana Press
Hervey T 2002 Mapping the contours of EU health law. European Public Law 69
Horton R 2000 Health and the UK Human Rights Act 1998. Lancet 356

Hunt M 1998 The horizontal effect of the Human Rights Act. Public Law 423

HMSO 1997 Rights brought home: The Human Rights Bill. Cm 3782

International Council of Nursing (ICN) Position statement regarding nursing and human rights (See http://www.icn.ch/pshumrights.htm accessed 17/05/02). Reprinted in Nursing Ethics 2001 8 (3): 272-3

Johnstone M J 1999 Bioethics: A nursing perspective, 3rd edn. W B Saunders & Harcourt, Merricksville, NSW

Kentridge S 1998 The incorporation of the European Convention on Human Rights. In: Constitutional reform in the UK: Practice and principles

Klug F 2000 Values for a godless age – The story of the United Kingdom's new bill of rights. Penguin Books, London

Klug F, Starmer K 2001 Incorporation through the front door: The first year of the Human Rights Act 1998. Public Law 65

Leaning J 2001 Health and human rights. British Medical Journal 322: 1435-1436

Lutzen K, Barbosa da Silva A 1996 The role of virtue ethics in psychiatric nursing. Nursing Ethics 3 (3): 202-11

Mann J M, Gruskin S, Grodin M A et al 1999 Health and human rights – A reader. Routledge, London

McGoldrick D 2001 The UK Human Rights Act 1998. International and Comparative Law Quarterly 90

Montgomery J 1992 Recognising a right to health. In: Beddard R, Hill D (eds) Economic, social and cultural rights: Progress and achievement. Macmillan, Basingstoke

Overs C, White R 2002 The European Convention on Human Rights, 3rd edn. Oxford University Press, Oxford

Rafferty A M, Robinson J, Eikan R (eds) 1997 Nursing history and the politics of welfare. Routledge, London

Sellman D 1997 The virtues in the moral edication of nurses: Florence Nightingale revisited. Nursing Ethics 4 (1): 3-11

Straw J, Boateng P 1996 Bringing rights home. Labour Party, London. Reprinted in EHRLR 71

United Nations General Assembly 1989 The Convention on the Rights of the Child

Wade H R W 2000 Horizons of horizontality. LQR 217

Whitty N, Murphy T, Livingstone S 2002 Civil liberties law. Butterworths, London

Wilkinson R, Caulfield H 2000 The Human Rights Act – A practical guide for nurses. Whurr Publishers, London

Zilgalvis P 2002 The European Convention on Human Rights and Biomedicine: Its past, present and future. In: Garwood-Gowers A, Tingle J, Lewis T (eds) Healthcare law: The impact of the Human Rights Act 1998. Cavendish, London

Websites

World Medical Association Resolution of Human Rights – http://www.wms.net/e/policy/20-2-90_e.html

Amnesty – http://www.amnesty.org

Human Rights Watch – http://www.hrw.org

Office of the High Commissioner for Human Rights – http://www.unhchr.ch

Physicians for Human Rights – http://www.phrusa.org

Liberty – http://www.liberty-human-rights.org.uk/mhome.html

Chapter 2

Rights and reproduction

Introduction

Nurses, midwives and health visitors provide information, counselling, care and treatment in relation to genetics, family planning, reproductive technologies, pregnancy, childbirth and neonatal care. Technological and research developments in these areas urge a consideration of some of the most profound and complex philosophical and legal issues. What, for example, is the moral and legal status of the embryo? What are the implications of pregnancy 'surveillance' techniques, of the new genetics and of artificial reproductive technologies for existing and future generations? Controversies have arisen in relation to single women who wish to reproduce (so-called 'virgin births'); to post-menopausal women who wish to have children; to sexual activity and reproduction in relation to persons who have learning disabilities; to women who wish to use the sperm of their incompetent or dead partners; to the anonymity of sperm donors; and to those couples who want to commission a surrogate. The 'right to choose' has also been challenged in relation to those women who elect to have Caesarean sections which are not medically indicated (provocatively labelled 'too posh to push' by the tabloid press).

The rhetoric of rights is rife in this area. Reproductive issues provide some of the most challenging and seemingly irresolvable rights conflicts. In relation to abortion, the right of the woman to control what happens in and to her body is often pitched against the rights of the foetus and/or the potential father. In relation to the provision of IVF, for example, the rights of the individual or couple are weighed against the interests of the potential child and of society as a whole. In relation to surrogacy the rights of the commissioning couple may, on occasion, conflict with the rights of the surrogate mother. The rights of the mother to determine the nature of childbirth have, in some instances, been challenged and/or overridden by professionals who claim to act in her 'best interests'. There is some dispute as to which individuals have rights (does the foetus have rights, for example?), as to what individuals and couples have a right regarding reproduction and whether a rights approach is an appropriate framework for the legal regulation of such issues. It has been pointed out, for example, that some feminists have expressed dissatisfaction with a rights approach to abortion and pregnancy in particular (Gibson in Chadwick 1998 p.5) and have argued that it pits the rights of the foetus against the rights of the mother, misrepresenting the mother-child relationship.

The NMC guidelines (Nursing & Midwifery Council 2002) which emphasise the importance of safeguarding and promoting the interests of individual patients and clients and serving the interests of society are as relevant to issues of reproduction as to other areas of health care. The NMC Code (2002) makes reference to the foetus in emphasising patient/client autonomy:

> '3.2 You must respect patients' and clients' autonomy – their right to decide whether or not to undergo any health care intervention – even where a refusal may result in harm or death to themselves of a foetus, unless a law orders to the contrary...'

Midwives have specific rules and a code of practice (NMC/UKCC 1998). In the Midwives Code of Practice (NMC/UKCC 1998) one of the responsibilities of the midwife is outlined as follows:

> 'As a midwife, you have a defined sphere of practice and you are accountable for that practice. The needs of the mother and baby must be the primary focus of your practice.'

'Mother and baby' is taken to be a reference 'to the mother and her unborn baby during the antenatal and intranatal periods and to the mother and baby during the period from the birth of the baby to the end of the postnatal period'. There is no explicit reference to the possibility that, in some situations, the needs (and rights) of mother and baby may conflict. The whole area of reproductive rights is accompanied by a vast literature. In this chapter we must necessarily be selective and have chosen some illustrations of human rights issues which impact on some selected aspects of reproduction and which nurses, in a number of roles and practice areas, may encounter.

A number of provisions of the European Convention of Human Rights which are included in the UK HRA 1998 appear to have relevance to reproduction. Those who believe that the foetus has the same moral status and rights as an adult may attempt to apply Article 2 (right to life) to abortion and embryo selection. Article 3 (prohibition of torture) may be applicable. At present the application of this Article in this area remains to be tested and raises a number of questions. Might it, for example, be argued that if the foetus is given protection under the ECHR then where a foetus feels pain late abortions should be prohibited? Or indeed that embryo research and genetic interventions are 'inhuman' and 'degrading'?

There is the prospect of the application of Article 8 (respect for private and family life). It might be argued that the law has no business interfering in private surrogacy arrangements or in situations where a husband/wife wishes to freeze sperm or eggs of incompetent partners. In the US case of *Eisenstadt v. Baird* (405 US 438 1972), Justice Brennan (Chadwick 1992 p.6) stated that:

'If the right of privacy means anything, it is the right of the individual, married or single, to be free from unwarranted governmental intrusion into matters so fundamentally affecting a person as the decision whether to bear or beget a child.'

Article 12 states that: 'Men and women of marriageable age have the right to marry and to found a family, according to the national laws governing the exercise of this right'. Chadwick (1992 p.4), writing prior to the incorporation of this article into British law through the Human Rights Act, points to the ambiguity of this right, asking: 'Does it imply that marriage is a necessary preliminary to the founding of a family?' and stating: 'Whether it could support a right for unmarried people to have children is a matter of controversy, as is the question as to whether it could provide a justification of an entitlement to reproduce by artificial means'.

Article 14 (prohibition of discrimination) may be applied to situations where, for example, the unmarried or homosexual are treated differently regarding entitlement to the rights above. Maclean (in Chadwick 1992 p.4) has noted that:

'whilst the state may have no general duty to facilitate reproduction through technology or the supply of a partner, once facilities are provided – for example through *in vitro* fertilisation and surrogacy programmes – to deny access on grounds of sexuality is to infringe the right on a discriminatory basis.'

As Article 14 relates to the violation of other HRA 1998 rights, where no absolute right to reproductive technology is made explicit, it is uncertain how this will be applied in the future. We now turn to some aspects of relevant legislation which impact on reproduction and to the context of rights in this area.

Before the enactment of the Human Rights Act 1998 there was already much legislation concerning health care issues at the beginning of life. Abortion was made a criminal offence in England by the Offences Against the Person Act 1861 (Sections 58 and 59). The Infant Life Preservation Act 1933 made it an offence to destroy the life of a child capable of being born alive. The rights of the foetus are also recognised tangentially through actions in negligence in relation to harm caused to the foetus in the womb leading, for example, to disability through the Congenital Disabilities (Civil Liability)

Act 1976. The scope of the Offences Against the Person Act 1861 which prohibits the supply of any 'poison or other noxious thing' with the intention of causing a miscarriage has recently been the subject of consideration in a case brought by The Society for the Protection of the Unborn Child (SPUC) to outlaw the 'morning-after' pill (*R (on the application of Smeaton) v Secretary of State for Health* [2002] 2 FLR 146). Whilst abortion remains illegal, the Abortion Act 1967 permits the termination of pregnancy if certain conditions are met. The Act also carries a conscientious objection clause which allows professionals to opt out of abortion. The Abortion Act was amended in 1990 by the Human Fertilisation and Embryology Act 1990. Under the legislation the so-called 'social' grounds for abortion under Section 1(1) are subject to a time limit of 24 weeks (see below for a fuller discussion of abortion). With technological advances which make it possible to maintain life at earlier stages, it is likely that this provision will be the subject of legislative consideration in the future.

The Human Fertilisation and Embryology Act 1990 regulates embryo research and aspects of reproductive technologies and techniques. The Human Fertilisation and Embryology Authority (HFEA) was set up under the 1990 Act. This body licenses clinics providing fertility treatment and embryo research (although it should be noted that not all such treatment is licensed under the legislation, e.g. where a woman is inseminated with her partner's sperm). The legislation also prohibits certain activities from being licensed under Section 3. The HFEA considers issues relating to human reproduction as they emerge, and consults widely about reproductive treatment and research issues which are particularly challenging. The Authority has undertaken consultation processes in relation to sex selection, the uses of ovarian tissue and, most recently, in relation to pre-implantation genetic diagnosis. The Surrogacy Arrangements Act 1985 regulates surrogacy in Britain, with non-commercial surrogacy permitted and payment of expenses allowed.

Reproductive rights have been the subject of much discussion at an international level. The 1994 International Conference on Population and Development in Cairo and the 1995 Fourth World Conference on Women in Beijing are credited with recognising the importance of human rights in relation to human reproduction (Cook & Fathalla 1998). The Cairo programme, building on the WHO definition of health, states that reproductive health:

'... implies that people are able to have a satisfying and safe sex life and that they have the capability to reproduce and the freedom to decide if, when and how often to do so. Implicit in this last condition are the rights of men and women to be informed and to have access to safe, effective, affordable and acceptable methods of family planning of their choice, as well as other methods of their choice which are not against the law, and the right of access to appropriate health-care services that will enable women to go safely through pregnancy and childbirth and provide couples with the best chance of having a healthy infant.'

The Beijing Declaration reaffirmed the definition of reproductive health as defined in Cairo and goes on to link human rights and reproduction explicitly:

> '[t]he human rights of women include their right to have control over and decide freely and responsibly in matters relating to their sexuality, including sexual and reproductive health, free of coercion, discrimination and violence. Equal relationships between women and men in matters of sexual relations and reproduction, including full respect for the integrity of the person, require mutual respect, consent and shared responsibility for sexual behaviour and its consequences.'

In Beijing, it was pointed out that 'reproductive rights embrace certain human rights that are already recognised in national laws, international human rights documents and other consensus documents' (cited by Cook & Fathalla 1998 p.2). It is not clear what might be claimed on the basis of Cairo and Beijing. There is evidence of positive and negative rights in relation to reproduction in these quotations. Where a negative right to reproduce is claimed, there is an expectation that the individual or couple will be free to reproduce without interference. Where a positive right to reproduce is stated, claims might be made for services which enable reproduction. The Cairo view of reproductive health includes a right to information, and access to family planning is implied but it is not clear if this could extend to reproductive technologies such as IVF. The Human Rights Act 1998 may potentially encompass both a negative and a positive rights based approach.

We turn now to some practice implications of rights in relation to reproduction.

The right to reproduce

Case 2a

> *Mona is thirty-eight, divorced and has a successful career in banking. She would very much like to be a mother but realises that she is too old to adopt. She had previously been advised that she would need IVF to conceive. She feels that she has much to offer as a parent, having the financial means to provide a good home for a child. She says that she is willing to go to court, if necessary, to argue for the right to reproduce.*

In 1978, the birth of the first 'test-tube baby' Louise Brown, signalled entry to a new era of reproduction. *In vitro* fertilisation (a process where sperm and eggs are fertilised in a petri dish and then placed in the uterus), is now fairly commonplace. During the 1998/9 period over 27,000 patients received IVF treatment in Britain and 6,450 live births resulted (18.2% of treatments) (HFEA 2000). The cost financially and emotionally is, then, high with treatment costing £5,000 to £10,000 and success being by no means guaranteed. Concerns regarding some of the legal and ethical issues resulting from the developments of modern reproductive technologies in the early 1980s led to the establishment by the Government of an inquiry, established in July 1982 and chaired by Dame Mary Warnock, with the following terms of reference:

'To consider recent and potential developments in medicine and science related to human fertilisation and embryology; to consider what policies and safeguards should be applied, including consideration of the social, ethical and legal implications of these developments; and to make recommendations.'

The Warnock Report was published in 1984. It recommended the introduction of new legislation to govern fertility treatment and embryo research and the creation of a new statutory licensing authority. The Report led to the passage of the Human Fertilisation and Embryology Act 1990. The Human Fertilisation and Embryology Authority (HFEA) was established under the 1990 Act. The HFEA issues a code of practice providing guidance to licensed clinics as to their provision of services for clients. The HFEA also provides information for potential patients about fertility services and details of clinics licensed for IVF.

Nurses have a number of roles to play in relation to IVF and other reproductive technologies. They may give information and/or direct individuals or couples to the HFEA for further information. Nurses may also be involved in counselling which is an important part of the care of those who have difficulty conceiving.[1] Nurses may act as advocates for women such as Mona should she/they feel unable to articulate her/their needs to the multi-disciplinary team. It may be that Mona needs to have an opportunity made available to explain her predicament and to locate the information and expertise necessary to make an informed choice. Nurses who work in fertility centres may also be involved in decision-making about access to treatment.

This short case study raises questions about criteria for access to IVF and about the rationale for the provision of IVF and other reproductive technologies. A number of arguments are presented in support of reproductive technologies. It has been argued that infertility is an illness; that the desire for a child is based on human biology; and that there is a right to reproduce (see Frith in Chadwick 1998). Counter arguments state that infertility is not a disease; that the desire for a child is not genetically determined; that there is no positive right to reproduce; and also that associated genetic screening may have undesirable consequences.

There is no consensus about the disease/illness status of infertility. Some women, like Mona perhaps, may argue that childlessness has had a negative effect on their mental health. If this is proven, the right to reproduce may then be linked to the right to health care. The Warnock Report (1985) acknowledged that infertility should be considered as any other 'malfunction':

1 There is some controversy as to whether this can be non-directive – See Peterson A. 1999 Counselling the genetically 'at risk': the poetics and politics of 'non-directiveness' in Health, Risk and Society 1, 2353-65.

'Medicine is no longer exclusively concerned with the preservation of life but with remedying the malfunctions of the human body. On this analysis, an inability to have children is a malfunction and should be considered in exactly the same way as any other... In addition the psychological distress that may be caused by infertility in those who want children may precipitate a mental disorder warranting treatment. It is, in our view, better to treat the cause of such distress than to alleviate the symptoms. In summary, we conclude that infertility is a condition meriting treatment.' (ibid p.9-10)

As for whether there is a biological or genetic basis for the desire for a child, again it is unlikely that there will be agreement. Mona might argue that her desire for a child does have a biological basis. For our purposes here the rights argument has most relevance. There is much rhetoric, as indicated above, regarding rights and reproduction. Article 8 and Article 12 may be read jointly to suggest that there is a 'right to reproduce'. But the extent to which reproductive rights can validly be regarded as being positive rights rather than negative rights may be questioned. When recently rejecting the claim of access to IVF services by a prisoner the Court of Appeal in *R (Mellar) v Secretary of State for the Home Department* [2002] QB13 held that:

'Article 12 does not confer on a man an absolute right at all times to be enabled to procreate.'

While there is much heated debate regarding the application of rights in this area there is comparatively less overt consideration of the issue of resources in relation to reproductive technologies. Fertility treatments are expensive and in the past there have been low success rates though more recent research suggests that the success rate is improving (Sunday Times 2002). As will be discussed in Chapter 6, health care resources are already stretched. Whilst respecting a negative right to reproduce is generally without direct cost (except perhaps in relation to the provision of child benefit and providing support for a couple with learning or other disabilities who decide to reproduce), a positive right to reproduce may entail a corresponding obligation to provide treatment to those who are infertile. There may also be additional costs should multiple births result from IVF. A statement from the HFEA in 2002 (http://www.hfea.gov.uk/forMedia/archived/15042002.htm accessed 15/07/02) stated that the Authority had no plans to compel fertility clinics to take out insurance to cover neonatal care should multiple births result. Most European countries, including Britain, allow a maximum of two embryos to be implanted and it was recently claimed that this may be too high as there is an increased risk of premature births and low birth weights with multiple births. The HFEA responded by saying that they were aware of this research but would continue with its guidance of two embryos. HFEA representative, Ann Furedi said:

'In Britain we are seeing a situation where doctors involved in IVF are really trying to minimise the risk of multiple pregnancy. At the same time they are facing pressure from patients who really want to maximise their chances of success through IVF.' (Henderson 2002)

The provision of fertility treatment is currently not universal and many couples will pay to have treatment privately. In considering Mona's case, what criteria might be used?

The HFE Act 1990 provides in Section 13(5) that:

'A woman shall not be provided with treatment services unless account has been taken of the welfare of any child who may be born as a result of the treatment (including the need of that child for a father), and of any child who may be affected by the birth.'

The HFE Authority sets out guidance regarding access to modern reproductive technologies. In Part 3 of the 2001 Code (HFEA 2001 Chapter 3) the first general obligation is stated as:

'3.1 Centres should take all reasonable steps to ensure that people seeking treatment and any children resulting from it have the best possible protection from harm to their health. Before providing any woman with treatment, centres must also take account of the welfare of any child who may be born or who may be affected as a result of the treatment.'

The Code goes on:

'3.3 In deciding whether or not to offer treatment, centres should take account both of the wishes and needs of the people seeking treatment and of the needs of any children who may be involved. Neither consideration is paramount over the other, and the subject should be approached with great care and sensitivity. Centres should avoid adopting any policy or criteria that may appear arbitrary or discriminatory.'

The HFEA does suggest 'factors to be considered' (HFEA 2001 p.16) and highlights the importance of the 'the welfare of the child'. Section 3.10 of the Code states:

'Centres should have clear written procedures to follow for assessing the welfare of the potential child and of any other child who may be affected. The HFE Act does not exclude any category of woman from being considered for treatment. Centres should take note in their procedures of the importance of a stable and supportive environment for any child produced as a result of treatment.'

Centres are asked to 'bear in mind' the commitment of the individual/couple, their ability to provide a 'stable and supportive environment' for a child, medical history, health, ages, any risk of harm and the effect of a new baby on existing children. As in the 1990 Act, the Code provides that the child's need for a father be considered. It provides that:

'Centres are required to have regard to the child's need for a father and should pay particular attention to the prospective mother's ability to meet the child's needs throughout their childhood. Where appropriate, centres should consider particularly whether there is anyone else within the prospective mother's family and social circle willing and able to share the responsibility for meeting those needs, and for bringing up, maintaining and caring for the child.' (HFEA 2001 p.17)

It is uncertain how a treatment centre would rule on the eligibility of someone like Mona. Although she does not have a partner, she appears to have family support and the financial means to provide for a child. In any case, doctors in the centres would make the decisions but there may be consultation with other professionals including nurses. There is, however, a question regarding the arbitrariness of access decisions as value judgements have to be made about appropriateness for parenthood. The BMA has taken the view that in difficult cases, doctors 'would benefit from the views of ethics committees' (BMA 1993 p.115). It is not the case, however, that an ethics committee will interfere with or override the decision of a doctor. A denial of IVF treatment was challenged in *R v Ethical Committee of St. Mary's Hospital, Manchester* [1988] 1 FLR 512. R was unable to conceive. Her application to adopt a child had been rejected because of her criminal record relating to prostitution and brothel keeping. She sought IVF treatment and her application was rejected by the consultant at the IVF clinic. He had become aware of the refused adoption and the reasons for this. Because of this and other reasons he refused the treatment. The hospital's infertility ethics committee took the view that the decision was for the medical team to make. R applied to the courts to oblige the committee to investigate the matter and to be heard before guidance or advice was given. Schiemann was of the view that the committee was an informal body and if it refused to give advice to a consultant in a particular case or did not reach a majority view he could not see that a court could compel it either to give advice or to enter into a particular investigation. He did emphasise however that:

'If the Committee had advised for instance that the IVF unit should in principle refuse treatment to anyone who was a Jew or coloured then I think that the court might well grant a declaration that this was illegal.'

In the case of *R v Sheffield HA ex parte Seale* [1994] 25 BMLR 1 a 36-year-old woman, S, was denied IVF treatment. The Health Authority had a policy of not providing treatment where the woman was over 35. It was said that there was a need to ration resources and that treatment was less effective in women over 35. This refusal to offer treatment was upheld by the courts. These cases demonstrate then that the courts are unwilling to intervene with discretionary decisions regarding the provision of fertility services.

In the case of Mona, above, whether she will be allowed access to IVF will depend on the criteria adopted in the particular centre and the view of the medical staff involved. Should she be refused treatment and bring legal proceedings, it is uncertain how the courts would rule post-HRA 1998. Her single parent status may not be sufficient to rule out access to IVF. The application of Article 8 and Article 12 may not be sufficient for the courts to rule in her favour.

A right to trace donor parents?

Case 2b

> *Miriam was born as a result of IVF and donor insemination. She now wants to trace her biological father.*

Currently, neither recipient parents nor resulting child have a right to know the identity of donors of sperm or eggs. This follows concerns expressed in the Warnock report that persons would not be prepared to come forward to donate gametes without the guarantee that they would not be able to be traced in later years (Warnock 1985). Section 31 of the 1990 Act requires the HFEA to maintain a register of information which has been obtained from licensed centres. This includes information that individuals may have been born consequent upon treatment services which were provided under the legislation. Section 31(3) enables persons aged over 18 to obtain specified information. Individuals may obtain information where they have been given a sufficient opportunity for counselling. Section 31(5) provides that regulations may specify what information is to be given. However, such regulation has to date not been made.

It has been argued that the Human Rights Act 1998 can be used to support a claim of access to donor information. Analogies can be drawn with the Children Act 1975 which provides that adopted children could obtain at the age of 18 a copy of their original birth certificate. In *Gaskin v UK* [1989] 1 FLR 167, the European Court of Human Rights held that Article 8 has the effect that 'everyone should be able to establish details of their identity as individual human beings'.

In *R (on the application of Rose) v Secretary of State for Health* [2002] WL 1446174; [2002] 2 FLR 962 Rose, an adult, and a child known as EM, who had both been born through the use of IVF with donated sperm, sought information about the sperm donor. They argued that the claim was justified due to Article 8 of the ECHR. They sought either identifying information or considerable non-identifying information which included blood type, medical history, social and family background, religion, skills and interests, occupation and willingness to be approached for further information. In the High Court Scott Baker J adjourned the majority of the issues pending the results of the Department of Health consultation. However he did hold that Article 8 was engaged here and stated that:

> 'Private and family life is a flexible and elastic concept incapable of precise definition. Respect for private and family life can involve positive obligations on the state as well as protecting the individual against

arbitrary interference by a public authority. Respect for private and family life requires that everyone should be able to establish details of their identity as individual human beings. This includes their origins and the opportunity to understand them. It also embraces their physical and social identity and psychological integrity. Respect for private and family life comprises to a certain degree the right to establish and develop relationships with other human beings. The fact that there is no existing relationship beyond an unidentified biological connection does not prevent Article 8 from biting.' (para 45)

He went on to say that it was understandable that such children should want to know their origins and that in view of today's much more open society:

'Secrecy nowadays has to be justified where previously it did not.' (para 47)

Moreover, he stated that Article 8 did encapsulate through ECHR jurisprudence (*Gaskin v UK* (1989) 12 EHRR 36) the incorporation of personal identity. Reference was also made to an individual's ability to establish his identity (*Johnstone v Ireland* (1987) 9 EHRR 303). There was the prospect that Rose and EM could argue that the Secretary of State should enact regulations which would enable further disclosure, however at this stage they could not make any statement as to whether or not it was the case that a declaration of incompatibility could be awarded.

While it was held that the action could be brought, a ruling will not be made until the government consultation on this issue has been completed. The Department of Health issued a consultation as to whether the requirement for donor anonymity should be maintained in 2001 ('Donor Information Consultation: Providing information about the donors of gametes and embryos' Department of Health (2001) http://www.doh.gov.uk/ gametedonors). Some studies have indicated that without anonymity donation levels would fall (Maclean & Maclean 1996). It appears that opinions on this issue are divided. The BMA recently voted against the removal of anonymity at their annual conference (contrary to advice from the BMA Medical Ethics Committee (The Times 2002)). However the HFEA recommended that there 'should be a move toward the removal of donor anonymity', although not retrospectively. Interestingly in Sweden legislation on artificial insemination enables identifying information regarding donors to be kept for a period of up to 70 years and there is a right to access information. The Swedish experience has been that while initially donation levels fell, this position then changed, with donation levels eventually reaching their original levels – although with those coming forward to be donors are now tending to be older and frequently married (Morgan & Lee 2001). The rights of the individuals/couples who have used donor gametes are also an issue. Infertility is a sensitive issue and parents may not want to inform their offspring that they have been born through the use of donor insemination. In February 2003 the health minister Hazel Blear stated that the government is to give persons born through sperm, egg and embryo donation the right to greater information (Dyer 2003). However the decision as to whether anonymity will be removed has been delayed in the light of concerns about the effect that removal of anonymity may have upon the supply of donors.

In Miriam's case, she is currently unable to trace her biological father. Challenges to the law on the basis of Articles 8 and 14 may, however, change this situation in the future.

The right to reproduce via surrogacy

Case 2c

> *Ellen and John would very much like to have a baby and seek advice from the fertility clinic at their local hospital. Ellen had to have an emergency hysterectomy when she was 21 so was unable to become pregnant. The couple had considered adoption but decided that, as far as possible, they would like a child of their own. They tell the nurse that they had searched the web and come across a website which offered surrogacy. The couple ask if this is legal and whether it is available on the NHS.*

Surrogacy has been described as 'the practice whereby one woman (the surrogate mother) carries a child for another person(s) (the commissioning couple) as the result of an agreement prior to conception that the child should be handed over to that person after birth' (Brazier et al 1997 p.3). 'Partial' surrogacy is the term used to describe the situation in which the surrogate mother is the genetic mother (i.e. her own egg used) and 'full' or 'host' surrogacy is where the commissioning couple have provided a fertilised embryo. The practice of surrogacy itself is lawful in England; however there is legal regulation of 'commercial surrogacy'. Surrogacy is regulated by the Surrogacy Arrangements Act 1985, which bans advertising and makes payments to third parties illegal, and by the Human Fertilisation and Embryology Act 1990. Section 2 of the 1985 Act makes it a criminal offence to make surrogacy arrangements on a commercial basis. Section 36 of the HFE Act 1990 amended the 1985 Act providing that 'no surrogacy arrangement is enforceable by or against any of the persons making it'. Thus surrogacy contracts are not enforceable in the courts – the surrogate mother cannot be compelled to hand over the child and the commissioning couple cannot be required to hand over or recover money paid to the surrogate mother. Section 2 of the 1990 Act also provides that 'the woman who is carrying or has carried a child as a result of the placing in her of an embryo or of sperm and eggs, and no other woman, is to be treated as the mother of the child'. This means that the surrogate mother, not the woman who is part of a commissioning couple, is regarded in law as being the mother. The commissioning couple can acquire parental rights through adoption. Alternatively, section 30 of the HFE Act permits a couple to be legally the parents of a child if certain conditions are met and the courts make an order. The conditions are that the child is genetically related to at least one of the commissioning couple; that the surrogate mother has given consent to the parental order no earlier than six weeks after the birth; that the commissioning couple are married to each other and over 18 years of age; that the commissioning couple have made the application within six months of the child's birth; that no money other than expenses has been paid unless authorised by a court; that the child is living with the commissioning couple; and that the couple usually live in the UK, Channel Islands or Isle of Man. In summary then, whilst surrogacy is permitted legally, surrogacy contracts are not legally enforceable, advertising is banned and payment to third parties is illegal.

In recent years, a good deal of controversy has surrounded surrogacy. In 1999 a British woman, Helen Beasley, who had agreed to be a surrogate mother for a Californian couple initiated legal proceedings against them as they had asked her to terminate the pregnancy when it was discovered that she was carrying twins. She refused and the couple then attempted to transfer their parental rights to another couple for £45,500 (BBC News 15/08/01). A gay couple were said to have made legal history when a US court gave them the right to be named on birth certificates as the parents of twins which were the result of a surrogacy arrangement. The British couple, Barrie Drewitt (a former nurse) and Tony Barlow (a dermatologist), had commissioned the surrogacy arrangement through a surrogacy agency in Los Angeles (Hartley-Brewer 1999). The couple are alleged to have paid £200,000 to an American surrogate mother. They are said to be planning a third child (Hall 2000).

Much of the controversy surrounding surrogacy relates to the payment of surrogates. In Britain, profit-making agencies are unlawful under the Surrogacy Arrangements Act 1985 but there are non-commercial organisations which offer support to couples who wish to enter into a surrogacy arrangement. COTS (Childlessness Overcome Through Surrogacy), which was founded in 1988, claims to have had 'over 450 successful surrogate births' (http://www.surrogacy.org.uk/FAQ4.htm accessed 20/07/02). A range of arguments are presented for and against surrogacy (see for example the Warnock Report (1985 Chap. 8)). There were, for example, concerns about 'commercialisation' and a 'trade' in babies; about potential damage to the child in the breaking of the bond with the carrying mother and in relation to his/her becoming aware that there was a financial aspect to the surrogacy arrangement; there were concerns about the risk of rejection of the baby due to disability or, as in the Beasley case, when more babies resulted than were desired; about either party changing their mind; and there were concerns about the exploitation of the surrogate mother and the risks which are involved in pregnancy. It has been argued that it is 'inconsistent with human dignity that a woman should use her uterus for financial profit and treat it as an incubator for someone else's child' (Warnock 1985 p.45). Arguments in favour of surrogacy relate to the fact that surrogacy should not be ruled out as it gives some couples the only chance of having a child which is genetically related to one or both of them. Further, it is suggested that surrogacy is altruistic and represents 'a deliberate and thoughtful act of generosity on the part of one woman to another' (ibid p.45).

So what impact might the European Convention and Human Rights Act 1998 make in relation to surrogacy? Could Ellen and John claim that they have a right to access surrogacy? The most relevant articles in relation to surrogacy are Articles 8 (right to respect for private and family life), 12 (the right to marry and found a family) and 14 (non-discrimination). It is, at least, possible that opponents of surrogacy might cite an argument which appeared in the Warnock Report (1985 p.45) and challenge on the basis of Article 3 (right to freedom from torture, inhuman or degrading treatment) – that is, that it is 'inconsistent with human dignity that a woman should use her uterus for financial profit and treat it as an incubator for someone else's child' (Warnock 1985 p.45). As yet, surrogacy cases have not been considered under the Human Rights Act 1998, however it is likely that the Act may be used by potential parents or by the surrogate mother and commissioning couple should one party wish to opt out of the arrangement. Article 8 protects individual autonomy in the private and public sphere. The right is qualified and must be weighed against, for example, the 'protection of health and morals, or for the protection of rights and freedoms of others'. As with other areas of reproduction, arguments that there is a positive right to a means of reproduction such as surrogacy, with demands that the health service bears the cost, seem unlikely to succeed. A question arises also as to what 'family' consists of in a surrogacy case as the arrangement is unconventional. In the case of *G v Netherlands* (1993) 16 EHRR CD 38, 'family life' was said to imply 'close personal ties in addition to parenthood'. Thus a sperm donor was unable to utilise the section to claim rights. It would seem that Ellen and John qualify in this respect. It has been suggested that Article 8 could 'provide support to a couple seeking to obtain custody of a child born of surrogacy' (Ramsey 2000 p.60). The same Article might also be used by a surrogate mother as the right to privacy can be said to apply to the right of a woman to use her body as she wishes (ibid p.60-61). It has also been suggested that a ban on payments might lead to another challenge:

> 'The banning of payments may therefore lead to an infringement of the commissioning parents' reproductive liberty, having the knock on effect of limiting reproductive choices to the fertile also. If intending parents, and women who might offer themselves as surrogates, are prevented from achieving their goals by the prohibition on payments envisaged by the Brazier Report, then arguably a case might be made that this amounts to a violation of Article 8.' (Ramsey 2000 p.61)

Article 12 discussed above in relation to the provision of IVF has been interpreted as, on the one hand, meaning that marriage is a necessary pre-requisite for founding a family and, more broadly, as meaning that 'no-one who wants a child should be denied the chance to have one, regardless of sexual orientation, age or anything else' (Bosseley et al 2000, cited by Ramsey 2000 p.54). It is uncertain as to what extent the English courts will be prepared to expansively interpret Article 12.

In October 1997, a consultation exercise 'Surrogacy – Review for the UK Health Ministers of current arrangements for payment and regulation' took place, led by Professor Brazier (Brazier 1998). Terms of reference included a consideration of payments (whether they should be allowed and on what basis); regulation (whether and how surrogacy should be regulated); and legislation (whether changes needed to be made to the Surrogacy Arrangements Act 1985 and the HFE Act 1990). The resulting report concluded that payment should cover only genuine expenses associated with the pregnancy; that agencies should be required to register and operate within a pre-determined Code of Practice, which would be supported by a new surrogacy act; and that sections of the HFE Act 1990 would be replaced by a new surrogacy act. Regarding the principles of the Code of Practice, it was concluded that the welfare of the child would be the paramount concern. It added 'surrogacy should remain an option of the last resort available only to couples where the intending mother's conditions renders pregnancy impossible or highly dangerous to her' (Brazier Report 1998 p.4-5). No legislative amendments have yet been made in the light of the Brazier report, nonetheless the prospect of a more comprehensive legislative review of this area may lead to this issue being revisited in the context of surrogacy.

The right to have a child of a certain kind

Case 2d

> Susan and Thomas are in their mid-thirties and now wish to try for a baby. One of Susan's brothers suffers from haemophilia and they have sought genetic counselling on the advice of their GP. On the basis of the discussion with the counsellor, they decide to opt for pre-implantation sex selection as only male children will be affected.

There has been debate not only about the right to reproduce but also about the right to have a healthy, perfect or 'designer' child. Developments in genetics offer potential parents the opportunity to find out about the genetic status, including the sex, of their potential child before implantation and prenatally. In December 2000 the HFEA and the HGC (Human Genetics Commission) set up a joint working party on pre-implantation genetic diagnosis (PGD) leading to a public consultation. The working party were against the use of PGD, stating that it should not be used deliberately to choose 'desirable' characteristics and also that it should not further disadvantage those who are disabled now or in the future. The HGC 'strongly' recommended the use of PGD only for 'specific and serious conditions' (see http://www.doh.gov.uk/hgc/business_publications_

statement_pgd.htm) Distinguishing specific and serious conditions from those less specific and serious is challenging.

Sex selection is regarded as controversial due to the potential for use for social as well as for medical reasons. In 1993 the HFEA carried out a consultation exercise to ascertain views about sex selection. They concluded that whilst it was acceptable for medical reasons, it was not so for social reasons. Medical reasons involve the use of sex selection techniques to prevent sex-linked diseases. There are some 200 such diseases usually affecting males, for example, colour blindness, haemophilia and muscular dystrophy. More generally, there has been debate about the acceptable conditions to warrant genetic testing. In their 1993 report, The Nuffield Council on Bioethics stated that the 'prime requirement' is that the condition was to be a serious disease (Nuffield 1993; Chadwick 1997). While many of the sex-linked disorders are undoubtedly 'serious' (such as haemophilia as in the case study), others (such as colour blindness, for example) seem less so. Social reasons for sex selection may be various. Some parents may want a 'balance' of sexes or it may be that cultural values result in a preference for one sex over another. The latter leads to the charge of 'designer babies' and discrimination. In some hospitals this has led to a decision not to tell parents the sex of the foetus as this may then become grounds for abortion.

There are two categories of sex selection. Primary sex selection is carried out before implantation and relates to two techniques: sperm sorting and timing of insemination. The former involves sorting sperm into that which carries the X chromosome (female) and that which carries the Y chromosome (male). It is this technique which has been offered by private clinics in London, Birmingham and Glasgow. Potential parents pay up to £3,500 for the service which sorts the sperm by spinning it at high speed. The success rate is said to be between 70 and 80% (The Observer 4/11/01). There have been reports of an American clinic which uses a sophisticated sperm sorting machine (MicroSort) system which has higher success rates – 92% for girls and 72% for boys (The Times 05/07/01). The second method of primary sex selection is premised on the belief that a child of a certain sex will result if the couple have sex at a certain period of the menstrual cycle. Secondary sex selection occurs after fertilisation either before the embryo is implanted (pre-implantation diagnosis – embryo cells are examined for X or Y chromosomes outside the body and then desired sex embryos selected) or after implantation (prenatal diagnosis). Nurses make an important contribution to this area, particularly at higher levels of practice, when they may work as specialists in genetics. They are likely to be involved in providing information and counselling.

There has been some opposition to sex selection at an international level. The Council of Europe in the Convention on Human Rights and Biomedicine provides in Article 14:

'The use of techniques of medically assisted procreation shall not be allowed for the purposes of choosing a future child's sex except where serious hereditary sex-related disease is to be avoided.'

Recent cases have brought the ethical and legal challenges of sex selection into sharp focus. A Scottish couple, Alan and Louise Masterton, have four boys and desperately want a girl after their three-year-old daughter was killed in a bonfire accident. They were refused access to sex selection techniques by the HFEA. They challenged the HFEA under human rights legislation – most notably Article 8. They considered, though ultimately did not pursue, an action before the European Court of Human Rights. Pre-implantation genetic diagnosis was at issue in the case of Raj and Hashana Hashmi from Leeds who asked the HFEA to permit IVF to produce a sixth child. Their fourth child, Zain, was diagnosed with beta thalassaemia major when he was five months old. He requires a blood transfusion every four weeks and an infusion of drugs for 12 hours five nights a week. He was not expected to live unless he received a stem cell or bone marrow transplant. Tests on the family to find a match failed so the parents had another baby in the hope that it would be a match. It was not. The couple then considered pre-implantation diagnosis and IVF. Using the couple's eggs and sperm, embryos would be produced and a single cell extracted from each. The cells would be sent to a laboratory in the US which has developed a test for thalassaemia. Affected cells would be discarded and those unaffected would be tissue-typed to find the best match for Zain. Two embryos that most closely match would then be implanted in Mrs Hashmi's womb. The intention was that after the child was born, blood cells taken from its umbilical cord, which is rich in stem cells, would be infused into Zain. It was reported that the HFEA was 'caught by surprise' as it was already carrying out a review of pre-implantation genetic diagnosis and had previously ruled out the selection of embryos for 'social, physical or psychological characteristics' but had not anticipated the scenario where embryos were 'selected not for their intrinsic merits but for their utility to another'. In December 2001 the HFEA announced its decision, 'in principle, to allow tissue typing to be used in conjunction with pre-implantation diagnosis for serious genetic disease' (http://hfea.gov.uk/whatsnew/newpress4.htm accessed 13/02/02). The HFEA gave the Hashmi's specific permission to pre-select a baby who will be a suitable donor for their son (Meek 2002). It was reported that 'at least six British couples' are preparing to seek permission to use genetic technology to pre-select a baby which will be a donor to help save the life of a sibling (Mayes & Waterhouse 2002). The HFEA was criticised for its ruling in the Hashmi case. The House of Commons Science and Technology Committee, for example, asserted that the HFEA should have consulted more widely on this issue (BBC News 'Designer baby' ruling condemned 18/07/02).

The HFEA's decision led to a High Court challenge by a pro-life campaigner, Josephine Quintavelle and the group CORE (Comment on Reproductive Ethics) (*R (on the application of Quintavelle) v HFEA* [2002] WL 31676428). It argued that the practice of tissue typing in such situations was not only ethically questionable but that in sanctioning it, the HFEA had acted beyond its powers. In the High Court Maurice Kay J commented that he had great sympathy for the family's position. However he held that the

HFEA was not empowered to sanction tissue typing because it was not an activity which fell within those sanctioned under section 2(1) of the Human Fertilisation and Embryology Act 1990. Section 2(1) provided that treatment services were to be defined as:

'medical, surgical or obstetric services provided to the public or a section of the public for the purposes of assisting women to carry children.'

In this particular instance the procedure was not something which was related to helping a person conceive or carry a child to term. He only gave brief consideration to arguments put before him on the basis of the parents' right to respect for private and family life under Article 8 and also to the right to life of their son under Article 2. He stated that he was of the view that there was no incompatability between the 1990 Act and the ECHR on this point. He noted that there was a margin of appreciation for Parliament on this issue and that:

'It seems that the activity which HFEA seeks to licence is unlawful in most if not all Convention countries.' (para 18)

The decision was overturned by the Court of Appeal on 8th April 2003 and the Hashmis are now able to seek treatment (http://news.bbc.co.uk/1/hi/health/2928655,stm). At the time of writing, the Appeal Court's reasoning was not available but it may be the case that the Human Rights Act has had a positive application in this area.

Clearly, the cases of the Mastertons and the Hashmis differ. In the first case, there is a wish to bring about a child of a certain sex for social reasons. In the second, the parents wish to have a child who is a genetic match and who will be a donor for a child who is likely to die without the donation. In the case of Susan and Thomas above, their reasons are medical and the condition for which they are requesting pre-implantation genetic diagnosis is a serious one, and thus thus there is a greater likelihood that the treatment will be sanctioned.

The potential for the use of the Human Rights Act in screening cases is undoubtably there. Nevertheless it is likely that in view of the controversy in this area generally any further judicial determinations are likely to be circumspect.

The right to stop pregnancy – the case of the minor and the morning-after pill

Case 2e

Jenny is 15 and comes to see the family planning nurse, Patricia, in her GP practice. She requests advice about the morning-after pill. She also says that she does not wish her parents to know. Patricia is uneasy about this as she has concerns regarding the administration of the morning-after pill.

There continues to be controversy and concern regarding early sexual activity and under-age pregnancies in Britain. Nurses who work in the community and in schools have to respond to the requests of young people for contraceptive advice. With expansion of the scope of practice, many nurses are now in a position to administer the morning-after pill under patient group directions. As with reproductive and genetic technologies it would appear that no absolute right to contraception can be claimed if someone is under age. The professionals must judge if the young person has 'sufficient maturity and intelligence'. The issue of conscientious objection is also relevant here as some professionals may believe that contraception is wrong. In this situation a referral must be made to a professionals who will provide appropriate contraceptive advice.

In 1985 the House of Lords ruled that a doctor may provide a girl under 16 with contraceptive advice in appropriate circumstances without the consent or knowledge of her parents (this principle will apply equally to other health care professionals) (*Gillick v West Norfolk and Wisbech AHA* (HL) 1985 [1985] 3 All ER 402 ML).

It was held that:

1 A girl under 16 had the legal capacity to consent to medical treatment, including contraceptive treatment, if she had sufficient maturity and intelligence to understand the nature and implications of such treatment.
2 The parents' right to determine such matters ended when the child achieved sufficient intelligence and understanding to make its own decision.
3 There might be exceptional circumstances when in the interests of the child's welfare a doctor might give contraceptive advice and treatment without the permission or even knowledge of the parents.
4 The doctor must be satisfied that
  a the girl understood his advice
  b he could not persuade her to tell or allow him to tell her parents
  c she was likely to have sexual intercourse without or without contraceptive treatment
  d unless she received such advice or treatment her physical or mental health was likely to suffer, and
  e her best interests required such advice or treatment without the knowledge or consent of her parents.

Recently the use of contraceptive devices has been the subject of legal challenge. While family planning organisations take the position that a woman is not pregnant until implantation, SPUC (the Society for the Protection of the Unborn Child) argued that pregnancy begins with fertilisation. Section 58 of the Offences Against the Person Act makes it an offence to procure a miscarriage. Section 1 of the Infant Life Preservation Act 1929 makes it an offence to destroy the life of a child capable of being born alive. Recently, SPUC brought an action for judicial review of the sale of 'emergency contraception' in pharmacies (*R (on the applicatin of Smeaton) v Secretary of State for Health* [2002] 2 FLR 140). It has been argued that the morning-after pill is a means of procuring a miscarriage and thus that prima facie its administration would contravene the Offences Against the Person Act 1861 which forbids the supply of 'any poison or other noxious thing' with the intent to induce a miscarriage. An offence is not committed under that Act however where the procedure is undertaken in accordance with the Abortion Act 1967. This raises the question of when the embryo/foetus begins to matter morally and when it can be said to have legal status and/or rights. This issue will be discussed in the next section. This challenge was not successful. In the High Court Mumby J made reference to a number of authorities in this area. In a series of earlier cases the courts emphasised that implantation was the crucial factor as to whether the Abortion Act 1967 is applicable. In *R v Price* [1968] 2 All ER 282 a doctor was charged with fitting a woman with an IUD with intent to procure a miscarriage. On appeal Sachs LJ said that the question for the jury was whether the doctor knew/believed her to be pregnant and intended to cause a miscarriage or whether he was fitting an IUD as a contraceptive device. In *R v Dhingra* (1991) a doctor was charged under Section 58 after he fitted his secretary with an IUD some 11 days after they had intercourse. The judge here withdrew the case from the jury. He held that: 'It is highly unlikely that any ovum became implanted and only at completion of implantation does an embryo become a foetus'. In the light of these earlier cases it was unsurprising that the challenge was unsuccessful.

Interestingly, this case was not argued on the basis of the European Convention of Human Rights. Mumby J made it clear that it was not part of his function to determine when life began. On the ECHR itself he commented that:

'No one has addressed me on any aspect of either the Human Rights Act 1998 or the European Convention for the Protection of Human Rights and Fundamental Freedoms. Thus Mr Gordon has not sought to argue that the fertilised ovum has a right to life under Article 2... Nor, on the other hand did Mr Parker or any of the others seek to argue that the right to respect for private and family life protected by Article 8 extends to confer the kind of privacy interest protected right to distribute and use contraceptives which has been recognised by the Supreme Court of the United States of America... No one has suggested that the 1967 Act is incompatible with the Convention...'

Munby J concluded:

'Decisions on such intensely private and personal matters as whether or not to use contraceptives, or particular types of contraceptives, are surely matters which ought to be left to the free choice of the individual. And, whilst acknowledging that I have had no argument on the point, I cannot help thinking that personal choice in matters of contraception is part of that 'respect for private and family life' protected by Article 8 of the Convention.'

This is important for the nurse for more than one reason. Section 4 of the Abortion Act 1967 provides a right to conscientious objection. However in the case of the morning-after pill the nurse would have no such statutory right in the light of Mumby's judgment as the Abortion Act is not applicable. Her only prospect in that situation would be to argue that under Article 9 her freedom of conscience and belief entitled her to a right to opt out and not to administer the pill to the girl.

The right to abortion

Case 2f

> *Chris works as a nurse in a university. On her way to her office, she is approached by a 19-year-old student, Rachel, who appears distressed. They go to the office where Rachel tells Chris that she is pregnant and that she wishes to have an abortion. They are interrupted by Ben, another student, who comes into the room. He says that he is the father of the child and does not wish Rachel to have an abortion.*

In the introductory section of this chapter we referred to the conflict of rights which arises in relation to reproduction. Here it appears that the rights of Rachel (to have control over her body) and Ben (to be a father) are in conflict. It can also be argued that the rights of the foetus (to life) are in conflict with Rachel's rights.

Thus far, we have not directly addressed the rights of the embryo/foetus. There is considerable debate in the ethical literature regarding the status of the foetus (see, for example, Singer 1994, Dworkin 1993 and Palmer 1999). At one end of the spectrum is the sanctity of life approach stating that human life is sacred and that the foetus is a human person (conservative position) and thus requiring specific safeguards. In contrast there is a liberal view which states that the 'foetus is in most if not all morally relevant respects like a piece of tissue or a bit of the human body' (Hursthouse 1987 p.47).

The 'mixed strategy view' is that the foetus has varying moral status. 'Initially it is, in most morally relevant respects, like a bit of tissue or an organ of the body. As it develops it gradually becomes, in most morally relevant respects, like a lower animal, then like a higher one, and in the later stages of its development it is, in most if not all morally relevant respects, like a baby, and hence on a par with fully-developed, normal adult human beings' (ibid p.65).

Pro-life groups adopt a conservative position in relation to the foetus/embryo and promote sanctity of life and right to life arguments. Pro-choice groups may advance an extreme liberal view and argue that the woman has the right to decide what happens in and to her body. The mixed strategy position resembles the current abortion law.

Embryo research guidelines are more restrictive (the HFEA Act 1990 S3(3)(a) prohibits keeping or using an embryo after the appearance of the primitive streak or after 14 days, whichever is earlier) with earlier stages of development having less protection than later stages. There is then no consensus regarding rights and the foetus/embryo. Conservatives are likely to argue that the foetus/embryo has the same rights as an adult, including the right to life. Extreme liberals may argue that the foetus/embryo does not have rights. Philosophers such as Hams (1985), for example, have argued that only persons have a right to life ('persons' require self-consciousness, rationality etc.) (see discussion by Gibson in Chadwick 1998 Volume 1). Mixed strategists are likely to take a sliding scale position – the more mature the foetus, the more it is entitled to rights.

In English law the courts have consistently confirmed that the foetus has no independent legal rights separate from that of the mother. In *Paton v BPAS* [1978] 2 All ER 987 Balcombe LJ stated: 'The foetus cannot, in English law, in my view, have any right of its own at least until it is born and has a separate existence from its mother.' (See also *A G Ref (No 3 of 1994)* [1996] QB 581 [1998] AC 245 and *Re MB* [1997] 2 FLR 426 (discussed earlier in the consent chapter).

Despite the rhetoric in the abortion debate English law does not recognise any right to abortion. Nonetheless, it may be lawful if certain conditions are met. Abortion is unlawful if not sanctioned by the 1967 Act. First, save in an emergency, abortion needs to be sanctioned by two medical practitioners. In making their decision considerable discretion is given to medical practitioners. For example, consider Section 1(1)(a), the 'social grounds'. This subsection sanctions abortion up to 24 weeks where it may result in physical or mental injury to the woman or to any child of the family. It is unclear as to what is meant by 'children of the pregnant woman's family'. Some suggestions have been made that here 'family' refers to social rather than biological family and that it also includes, for example, adopted children. The statute also does not make clear at what point the time limit of 24 weeks actually runs from.

The other provisions under the Act are not subject to the time limit provision. Section 1(b) relates to the situation in which the abortion is 'necessary to prevent grave/permanent injury to the physical or mental health of the woman'. This ground was inserted by the HFE Act 1990. As has been noted by Kennedy and Grubb (2000) this provision does not require the doctors to balance out the risks between continuation of the pregnancy and the risk of the abortion being undertaken (ibid p.1423). It has also been suggested by Kennedy and Grubb (2000) that termination is necessary because it is actually the only course of action available in that situation to avoid that risk to the woman. Section 1(c) sanctions abortion in a situation in which there is a risk to the life of the woman. This again is a balancing provision between the risk of the pregnancy's continuation against the risk to the woman's life. Section 1(1)(d), which again sanctions abortion until birth, relates to handicaps. During debates on the Act there was some attempt to clarify what constitutes 'serious handicap'. However, this is still undefined.

A further difficulty with this Section is that there is no definition of what constitutes a 'substantial risk' of handicap in such a situation. This is particularly problematic in that it is frequently not possible to detect from prenatal screening the degree of handicap/disability which the foetus is suffering. Do these limitations infringe the ECHR, through for example the application of Article 3 and Article 8?

Stauch (2001) notes that the existing legislation is problematic due to the fact that the grounds for abortion are vague, leaving considerable discretion to the clinician. In addition there is considerable variation in access to NHS abortions in the country (Sheldon 1997). Stauch comments that 'such legislatively inspired arbitrariness is likely now to fall foul of the Human Rights Act 1998' (Stauch 2001 p.263). It will be interesting to see how this will operate against the fact that, as Stauch himself notes in an earlier case, the European Commission have held that 'Art 8(1) cannot be interpreted as meaning that pregnancy and its termination are, as a principle, solely a matter of the private life of the mother' (*Bruggemann and Scheuten v Germany* (1981) 3 EHRR 408).

What about Ben's rights in this situation? The nature/extent of the father's rights in the abortion process were extensively considered in *Paton v BPAS* [1978] 2 All ER 987. A husband sought and was refused an injunction to prevent his wife obtaining an abortion. He took his case to the European Commission on Human Rights claiming that Article 8, the right to respect for family life, enabled him to obtain an injunction. The Commission set out three alternative approaches: first, that Article 2 does not apply; second, that it does confer some rights but these are overborne by the interests of the mother in the early stages of pregnancy; third, that Article 2 gave the foetus a right equivalent to that of the adult. The Commission held that:

> 'The life of the foetus is intimately connected with, and cannot be regarded in isolation from, the life of the pregnant woman. If Art 2 were held to cover the foetus and its protection were, in the absence of any express limitation, seen as absolute, an abortion would have to be considered as prohibited even where the continuance of the pregnancy would involve a serious risk to the life of the pregnant woman. This would mean that the 'unborn life' of the foetus would be regarded as being of a higher value than the life of the pregnant woman.'

The Commission did not take either the first or the second position and say whether Article 2 applied to the foetus but they did say that the father had no right to be consulted. They stated that in so far as there was an interference of his rights under Article 8 they were justified under paragraph 2 because these were necessary to safeguard the rights of another person.

This approach was confirmed in the English courts in *C v S* [1988] QB 135 in the context of an unmarried couple. C wanted to stop his former girlfriend having a termination. The issue here revolved around whether the abortion itself was illegal. The foetus was 18 weeks old. The claim failed on these grounds. However, in the Court of Appeal, Lord Donaldson said that even had they had found in favour of C on other issues they would have given considerable weight to the judgment of Baker in *Paton v Trustees of the BPAS*:

> 'not only would it be a bold and brave judge who would seek to interfere with the discretion of doctors acting under the [Abortion Act 1967] but I think that he would really be a foolish judge who would try to do any such thing, unless possibly there is clear bad faith and an obvious attempt to perpetrate a criminal offence.'

In the case of Rachel and Ben, based on existing law, Rachel cannot be said to have a right to abortion as no such right exists. If, however, doctors conclude that the pregnancy will jeopardise her physical or mental health an abortion might be permitted. Previous cases suggest that Ben does not have rights in relation to the continuation of the pregnancy. If he did then this would, of course, compromise Rachel's right to decide. In relation to the HRA 1998 an application to the courts might be made on the basis of the foetus's right to life (Article 2). However, as noted above, the ECHR has not in the past taken such an approach. Also, Article 2 (if accepted) might be countered by Article 3 (subjecting a woman to a pregnancy she did not want might be considered inhuman and degrading). On the other hand, Article 3 might be related to the foetus to be aborted. Article 8 (right to respect for private and family life) was argued unsuccessfully in a previous similar case.

The nurse in the case study is obviously in a difficult position. The nurse will need to be aware of the boundaries of confidentiality in a case such as this (see privacy chapter).

Rights, consent and reproduction

Case 2g

> *Peter is 28 years old and is a patient on the intensive care unit. He has been involved in a road traffic accident and has suffered a serious head injury. His wife, Clare, visits regularly and tells staff that they had planned to have a family. When she is told that Peter's prognosis is poor, she asks nurses how she might go about extracting and freezing some of Peter's sperm.*

Peter is unconscious. Following the House of Lords decision in *Re F* [1990] 2 AC 1 procedures can only be undertaken on incompetent adults on the basis of necessity where it is in their best interests to do so. Best interests is a decision taken by reference to clinical judgement, though recently the courts have been prepared to take a somewhat broader approach (see Chapter 3). The relatives have no legal status to take the decision on behalf of the incompetent adult. The legality of the removal of sperm in such a situation is highly questionable and it is likely that such a removal would be a battery. The issue of posthumous use of sperm arose in the Diane Blood case (*R v Human Fertilisation and Embryology Authority ex parte Blood* [1997] 2 All

ER 687) (Lee & Morgan 1997). Her husband, Stephen Blood, developed meningitis. While in a coma, sperm was taken from him. The 1990 Act did not allow his wife to use his sperm for IVF treatment in England after his death as the sperm was taken when Mr B was unconscious and there had therefore been no prior consent before death. Instead his wife sought to have the sperm exported to Belgium. The HFEA rejected this on the basis that consent according to the legislation had not been given. This would be a major difficulty here as Peter has not had the opportunity to give his consent for the use of the gametes and the procedure could be a battery. Mrs Blood sought to have the sperm exported to Belgium so that she could undergo treatment in that jurisdiction. It was held that her free movement rights under EU law (Articles 59 and 60 EC Treaty) were a relevant factor which the HFEA should have taken into consideration. The matter was remitted to HFEA for reconsideration. Ultimately they granted her permission to export the sperm outside the jurisdiction and she later gave birth to a son, Liam. This is however an exceptional case and the legality of the removal of the sperm was never fully addressed in the case. A more likely approach is that the court would not sanction use.

The question of posthumous conception is controversial. It was raised again recently when it was reported that Mrs Blood was pregnant for a second time, again having received treatment in Belgium (Feb 2002). She has recently given birth to a second baby which was again conceived using sperm from her dead husband (BBC News 19/07/02). In such a situation, posthumous conception, the right to reproduce can be seen in conjunction with the issues around the welfare of the child and the need of the child for a father. These considerations are already highlighted in Section 13(5) of the 1990 Act discussed earlier. Article 8 and Article 12 are relevant in this context. In particular, what is the application of Article 12 and the right to marry and found a family? The ethical boundaries here are complex. A further issue in such a situation is that, according to Section 28(6) of the Act, any child born posthumously using treatment licensed under the Act will be legally fatherless, thus the birth certificate of Diane Blood's son Liam does not make any reference to his father Stephen. This position has been criticised.

A review was established following the Blood case to examine the issue of consent, with Professor Shelia McLean as chair (McLean 1997-8). It recommended that in cases such as Mrs Blood's, the father's name should be added to the birth certificate retrospectively. In summer 2000 the Government announced that they were intending to take this recommendation forward, but then did not do so. In 2000 Debra Shipley MP herself introduced a ten minute rule bill with the intention of amending Section 28. The Human Fertilisation and Embryology Bill 2000 provided that in a situation of posthumous pregnancy where the couple had been married/living together or otherwise receiving treatment services together the deceased man could be named as the father. Diane Blood then went to court to challenge the situation under the Human Rights Act. In February

2003 in the High Court lawyers for the Secretary of State for Health Alan Milburn conceded that the existing law was incompatible with the ECHR. This paves the way for a change in the law in this area. The judge, Sullivan J, was critical of the Department of Health having allowed the case to come before the court at all (http://bbc.uk.uk/hi/health/ 2807707.stm). A private members bill, The Human Fertilisation and Embryology (Deceased Fathers) Bill 2002, has been introduced with the aim of amending the law in this area and at the time of writing has been given a second reading and sent to standing committee.

This case brings reproductive rights into sharp focus and highlights the possibility that nurses in general practice may also have to grapple with the most profound issues. In the case of Peter and Clare, a nurse would be advised to consult with the multi-disciplinary team and to recommend the involvement of the Trust lawyer, as the legality of following Clare's wishes is highly questionable.

Conclusion

As evidenced in the discussion of some of the many reproductive and genetic issues which have emerged in health care in recent years, a rights discourse by itself seems ill-equipped to respond to these most challenging of issues. The rights of potential or actual mother, father, surrogate mother, potential child, existing children and the interests of society and future generations are sometimes at odds with each other.

The law as it stands bestows no absolute rights regarding reproduction. Access to services and treatments are generally at the discretion of health care professionals. Whilst doctors may have the last word, nurses will often be involved in such discussions. Research and technological developments in reproduction and genetics are continuing apace. If the recent press reports regarding extra-uterine pregnancies are actualised it is inevitable this will lead us to reconsider the boundaries and applicability of rights discourse in this area. In particular it will require rethinking male reproductive rights both in terms of access to reproduction and in terms of control over the foetus during pregnancy. A recent report of the 'world's first womb transplant' (Bosseley in The Guardian 7/03/02) also signals the possibility that, at some future time, surrogacy may be unnecessary. The rights and status of the foetus itself will also need to be reconsidered. We have considered some of the implications of specific HRA 1998 articles in relation to reproduction – Article 2 (right to life); Article 3 (prohibition of torture); Article 8 (respect for private and family life); Article 12 (right to marry and found a family) and Article 14 (prohibition of discrimination). Thus far these have, for the most part, not succeeded in bringing about significant changes in existing law but challenges will continue.

The challenges for law in terms of regulating technological developments will have a profound impact on existing and future generations.

The foreword to the Warnock Report (1985 p.2-3) states:

'There must be some barriers that are not to be crossed, some limits fixed, beyond which people must not be allow to go... Barriers, it is generally agreed, must be set up; but there will not be universal agreement about where these barriers should be placed. The question must ultimately be what kind of society can we praise and admire? In what sort of society can we live with our conscience clear?'

Warnock in her recent book 'Making Babies' (Warnock 2002) illustrates the difficulty of the establishment of barriers 'not to be crossed' in this area forcibly by highlighting that in many of the issues which were discussed in the Warnock Report, such as access to information about sperm donors and cloning, she now takes a different view. She has called for a Royal Commission to be established to redraft the Human Fertilisation and Embryology Act 1990 (http://news.bbc.co.uk/1/hi/health). The House of Commons Select Committee on Science and Technology have also suggested that the law in this area should be the subject of reconsideration (HC 2002).

In relation to reproductive and genetic developments the frontiers will continue to be pushed forward and it is of crucial importance that nurses are well acquainted with the ethical and legal dimensions of these developments.

References

BBC News 'Surrogate fights to stop twins sale' 15/08/01
    (http://news.bbc.co.uk/hi/english/health/newsid_1491000/1491926.stm)
BBC News 'Plea from sperm donor children' 22/05/02
BBC News 'Designer baby ruling condemned' 18/07/02
    (http://news.bbc.co.uk/hi/english/health/newsid_2134000/2134314.stm
    accessed 10/07/02)
BBC News 'Court win for donor sperm children' 26/07/02
BBC News 'Couple denied designer baby' 01/08/02
Bosseley S 2002 Surgeons hail world's first womb transplant. The Guardian
    07/03/02
Bosseley S 2002 Judge rejects ban on morning-after pill. The Guardian 19/04/02
Brazier M, Golombok S, Campbell 1997 Surrogacy – Review for the UK Health
    Ministers of current arrangements for payments and regulations. Consultation
    Document and Questionnaire
Brazier M 1998 Surrogacy – Review for the UK Health Ministers of current
    arrangements for payments and regulations. Cm 4068
British Medical Association 1993 Medical ethics today: Its practice and philosophy
    BMJ Publishing Group, London
Chadwick R 1992 Ethics, reproduction and genetic control. Routledge, London
Chadwick R 1997 Genetic screening: Ethical and philosophical perspectives.
    Euroscreen Final Report
Cook R J, Fathalla M F 1998 Duties to implement reproductive rights beyond
    Cairo and Beijing. Nordic Journal of International Law 67 (1): 1-16

Department of Health 2001 Donor information: Providing information about
    sperm, egg and embryo donors
Dworkin R 1993 Life's dominion – An argument about abortion and euthanasia.
    Harper Collins, London
Dyer C 2003 Egg or sperm donation children will be entitled to more information.
    BMJ 1st February; 326: 240
Frith L 1998 Reproductive technologies overview. In: Chadwick R (ed)
    Encyclopedia of applied ethics volume 3. Academic Press, San Diego
Gibson S 1998 Abortion. In: Chadwick R (ed) Encyclopedia of applied ethics
    volume 1. Academic Press, San Diego
Hall S 2000 Gay pair plan a third baby. The Guardian 01/06/00
Harris J 1985 The value of life. Routledge, London
Hartley-Brewer J 1999 Gay couple will be legal parents. The Guardian 28/10/99
Henderson M 2002 IVF clinics warned over dangerous multiple births
    (http://www.timesonline.co.uk/printFriendly/0,,1-2-344032,00.html)
House of Commons Select Committee on Science and Technology 2002
    Developments in human genetics and embryology HC 791
Human Fertilisation and Embryology Authority 2001 Code of Practice, 5th edn.
    HFEA, London
Human Fertilisation & Embryology Authority 2002 Press Release: HFEA statement
    on the cost of multiple births resulting from IVF
    (http://www/hfea.gov.uk/forMedia/archived/15042000/htm accessed
    15/07/02)
Hursthouse R 1987 Beginning lives. Blackwell in association with the Open
    University, Oxford
Kennedy I, Grubb A 2000 Medical law. Butterworths, London
Maclean S, Maclean M 1996 Keeping secrets in assisted reproduction. Child and
    Family Law Quarterly 8 (6): 243
Mayes T, Waterhouse R 2002 Six couples in queue for designer babies. The Sunday
    Times 24/02/02
McLean S A M 1997-8 Review of the common law provisions relating to the
    removal of gametes and of the consent provisions in the Human Fertilisation and
    Embryology Act 1990. Department of Health, London
Meek J 2002 Designer baby gets go-ahead. The Guardian 23/02/02
Morgan D, Lee R 1997 In the name of the father - ex parte Blood dealing with
    novelty and anomaly. Modern Law Review 40: 60
Morgan D, Lee R 2001 Human fertilisation and embryology: Regulating the
    reproductive revolution. Blackstone Press, London
Nuffield Council on Bioethics 1993 Genetic screening: ethical issues.
Nursing and Midwifery Council 1998 Midwives Code of Practice. NMC, London
Nursing and Midwifery Council 2002 Code of Professional Conduct. NMC,
    London
Palmer M 1999 Moral problems in medicine – A practical coursebook. The
    Lutterworth Pres, Cambridge
Ramsey J 2000 Regulating surrogacy – A contravention of human rights? Medical
    Law International 5: 45-64
Singer P 1994 Rethinking life and death – The collapse of our traditional ethics.
    Oxford University Press, Oxford
Stauch M 2001 Pregnancy and the Human Rights Act 1998. In: Garwood-Gowers
    A, Tingle J, Lewis T (eds) Healthcare law: The impact of the Human Rights Act
    1998. Cavendish, London

Sunday Times 2002 Abortion pill to be offered in clinics. The Sunday Times 07/07/02

Warnock M 1985 A question of life – The Warnock report on human fertilisation and embryology. Basil Blackwell Ltd, Oxford

Warnock M 2002 Making babies. Oxford Univesity Press, Oxford

Chapter 3

Human rights and consent to treatment

Introduction

Consent to treatment is a fundamental principle of English law. The principle of consent recognises the need to respect the autonomy of the individual patient. This is also recognised in the Nursing and Midwifery Council Code of Professional Conduct (2002) which states:

'3.1 All patients and clients have the right to receive information about their condition. You must be sensitive to their needs and respect the wishes of those who refuse or are unable to receive information about their condition. Information should be accurate, truthful and presented in such a way as to make it easily understood. You may need to seek legal or professional advice or guidance from your employer in relation to the giving or withholding of consent.'

Whilst there are many guidelines emphasising consent, the practice of consent is complex.

- Who can consent and in what situations?
- What constitutes valid consent in law?
- What do patients have to be told about the boundaries of consent?

The changing context of health care should be considered here. Patients are no longer passive recipients of information and now have access to more information than previously, from a far larger number of outlets – through the NHS (NHS Direct, for example) and also non-NHS (from the media, internet etc.) A number of Articles contained in the European Convention of Human Rights can be seen as being applicable in relation to consent to treatment.

- Article 2 (right to life) – might have a bearing on consent if patients/clients are not adequately informed about the risks of surgery or other treatments.
- Article 3 (prohibition of torture) – could apply if patients/clients are coerced into treatments or activities which they think are degrading or inhuman. An example might be electro-convulsive therapy where the consent of the patient has not been freely given.
- Article 5 – the right to liberty and security of the person.
- Article 8 (right to respect for private and family life) – as has been discussed elsewhere this is fundamentally respectful of autonomy. This principle underpins consent.
- Articles 9 (freedom of thought, conscience and religion) and 10 (right to freedom of expression) may support patients/clients in refusing interventions on the basis of culture or religion.
- Article 12 (right to marry and to found a family) – perhaps in relation to those with learning disabilities who may wish to refuse contraception or sterilisation.
- Article 14 (prohibition of discrimination) – might apply if, for example, there is differential treatment in the respect given to the refusal of treatment by children and adults.

We now turn to some of the more specific implications of rights in relation to consent in health care.

Consent is a principle which is inherent in relation to respect for the autonomy of the individual. It is integral to many major declarations of patient rights. English law requires that, before a patient is treated, his consent must be obtained. To treat without having obtained valid consent may give rise to liability in battery or to a criminal prosecution for common law assault/battery, or in the case of more serious surgical invasion, an offence under the Offences Against the Person Act 1861 for actual or grievous bodily harm (McHale 2002).

Consent is an area which has come under considerable scrutiny in recent years – in particular through the Bristol Inquiry Report (Kennedy et al 2001).

The Kennedy Report into the events at Bristol Royal Infirmary gave considerable consideration to questions regarding consent to treatment in the section of the report entitled 'Respect and honesty' (Kennedy et al 2001). The recommendations can be regarded as enhancing and reinforcing good practice in relation to consent. The Bristol recommendations also remind us that consent is not just applicable to surgical procedures, but relates to all activities that involve 'touching'. This includes many nursing procedures, such as providing assistance with washing and dressing, moving and handling, taking blood pressure and applying dressings. The Bristol Inquiry report also emphasised that consent can be best regarded as a process. It states that:

> '24. The process of informing the patient, and obtaining consent on a course of a treatment should be regarded as a process and not a one-off event consisting of obtaining a patient's signature on a form.
>
> 25. The process of consent should apply not only to surgical procedures but all clinical procedures and examinations which involve any form of touching. This must not mean more forms: it means more communication.
>
> 26. As part of the process of obtaining consent, except when they have indicated otherwise, patients should be given sufficient information about what is to take place, the risks, uncertainties, and possible negative consequences of the proposed treatment, about any alternatives and about the likely outcome, to enable them to make a choice about how to proceed.'

The Government in their response to the Bristol Inquiry Report have stated that they endorse this new guidance and confirm the principle that consent is a process and that the principle of consent is applicable to all clinical procedures – not simply to surgery. Moreover that 'patients should be given sufficient information about what is to take place, the risks, the uncertainties and possible negative consequences of the proposed treatment, about any alternatives and about the likely outcome, to enable them to make a choice as to how to proceed' (Department of Health 2001a).

Following the Bristol Royal Infirmary Inquiry, Health Secretary Alan Milburn, in a statement to the House of Commons responding to the Bristol Inquiry, commented that 'informed consent must be a cornerstone of a modern health service' (http://www.doh.gov.uk/bristolinquiryresponse/statement.htm). Subsequently the Department of Health followed Kennedy's recommendations and issued a 'Reference Guide to Examination and Treatment' (2001b) and new model consent forms (http://www.doh.gov.uk/consent). The issue of information and consent is considered below.

Who has the capacity to give consent? Adult patients are generally presumed to have capacity to make clinical decisions, however this presumption of capacity may come under challenge in the clinical situation. This may arise because the adult in question has a degree of mental disability. Alternatively the capacity question may arise in a situation in which a person who otherwise would have been regarded as being competent rejects the treatment options proposed. In such a situation there is a temptation to override the refusal on the basis that the person lacks capacity. In *Re C* [1994] 1 All ER 819 the court upheld the right of a 68-year-old person with paranoid schizophrenia with gangrene in his foot to prevent his foot being amputated in the future without his express written consent. Mr Justice Thorpe suggested a three-part test to determine capacity:

'... first, comprehending and retaining treatment information, secondly, believing it and thirdly, weighing it in the balance to arrive at a choice.'

The test was restated in *Re MB* [1997] 2 FLR 426. Here a woman with a needle phobia agreed to a Caesarean section, but repeatedly refused an anaesthetic prior to the operation. Butler Sloss LJ held that a person is not capable of making a decision where

'(a) the person is unable to comprehend and retain the information which is material to the decision, especially as to the likely consequences of having or not having the treatment in question; and

(b) the patient is unable to use the information and weigh it in the balance as of the process of arriving at a decision.'

In the case of the child and adolesecent there are further difficulties both in ascertaining whether the child has rights to give consent themselves but also and more particularly as to whether the child has the right to refuse clinical procedures. These issues are returned to below. The right to consent is circumscribed at present in law because there is no right to compel what treatment you seek. Some of these issues are explored further in relation to resources in Chapter 6 below.

The right to informed consent

Case 3a

> *Sarah is 78 and has been admitted to hospital for a hip replacement. Shortly after she arrives on the ward, a junior doctor arrives and announces that he is there to 'consent' the new admission for theatre the following morning. Later, Sarah asks the nurse for more information about the nature of the surgery, the name of the surgeon and the number of successful operations performed.*

What then are the implications for Sarah and the nurses involved in her care?

Health care professionals can certainly not be regarded as simply the imparters of information, while patients are not simply passive recipients. The internet and the media have contributed to patients being far more aware of the choices available to them and also more fearful of the risks that may arise from clinical procedures.

To ensure that there is no liability in battery here there must be disclosure of the broad nature of the procedure to be undertaken (*Chatterson v Gerson* [1981] 1 All ER 257). There should also be disclosure of certain consequent risks of clinical procedures and failure to do so may result in liability in negligence. However, English law has never required consent to be 'informed' consent as is recognised in other jurisdictions such as the USA/Canada (*Reibl v Hughes* [1980] 2 SLR 800; *Canterbury v Spence*, 1972). Instead, in *Sidaway v Bethlem Royal Hospital Governors* [1985] 1 All ER 673, Lord Diplock stated that the level of information disclosed should follow the standard used to determine whether clinical practice is negligent, namely that of a responsible body of clinical practice, adhering to the Bolam standard or test (*Bolam v Friern Hospital Management Committee* [1957] 2 All ER 118). In contrast Lord Scarman favoured a prudent patient test akin to the approach taken in other jurisdictions. Lord Bridge thought that, while the disclosure test was fundamentally one of professional practice, if there was some disagreement between clinicians then the court may resolve this. Also he stated that it may be negligent not to reveal a serious risk such as a ten per cent risk of a stroke. Lord Templeman was of the view that 'special' risks should be disclosed. Interestingly while the other law lords in *Sidaway* took slightly differing approaches, the Diplock approach was followed in subsequent court decisions (*Gold v Haringey Health Authority* [1987] 2 All ER 888; *Blyth v Bloomsbury AHA* (decided in 1987 but reported in [1993] 4 Med LR 151)).

Over time, however, the professional practice standard itself has begun to alter, and the trend today – which is arguably influenced at least in part by the fear of litigation – is towards enhanced disclosure of information to patients. The Courts have indicated that they are no longer prepared to necessarily accept the approach taken by one body of professional opinion. In *Smith v Tunbridge Wells* [1994] 5 Med LR 334 the judge held that the failure to warn – in this case concerning the prospect of a rectal prolapse – was not 'reasonable nor responsible' and was consequently negligent even though there was a body of professional opinion which supported the approach taken by the surgeon. This was however only a decision at first instance. However more recently there have been signs that the judiciary may be prepared to take a close look at the professional practice standard. In *Bolitho v City of Hackney HA* [1988] AC 232 Lord Browne Wilkinson stated that:

> 'In particular where there are questions of assessment of the relative risks and benefits of adopting a particular medical practice, a reasonable view necessarily presupposes that the relative risks and benefits have been weighed by the experts in forming their opinions. But if in a rare case, it can be demonstrated that the professional opinion is not capable of withstanding logical analysis, the judge is entitled to hold that the body of opinion is not responsible or responsible. I emphasise that in my view it will be very seldom right for a judge to reach the conclusion that views genuinely held by a competent medical expert are unreasonable.'

In this case Lord Browne Wilkinson distanced himself from disclosure of risk – however an approach more critical of clinical practice has been taken by the courts in subsequent cases. In *Pearce v Bristol NHS Trust* [1999] PIQR P53(CA) Lord Woolf stated that:

'if there is a significant risk which would affect the judgment of a reasonable patient then in the normal course it is the responsibility of a doctor to inform the patient of that significant risk, if the information is needed so that the patient can determine for him or herself as to what course that s/he should adopt.'

While on the facts of that particular case the plaintiffs failed to establish negligence it can be seen as a further step towards a broader duty of disclosure upon clinicians (Grubb 1999).

Nonetheless there is a real difference between making information available and that information being effectively communicated to the patient. The Bristol report and its recommendations need to be seen in the context of these developments. The report makes a number of specific recommendations in relation to patient information. It states, for example:

'4. Information about treatment and care should be given in a variety of forms, be given in stages and be reinforced over time.

5. Information should be tailored to the needs, circumstances and wishes of the individual.

6. Information should be based on the current available evidence and include a summary of the evidence and data in a form that is comprehensible to patients.

7. Various modes of conveying information, whether leaflets, tapes, videos or CDs should be regularly updated, and developed and piloted with the help of patients.'

What appears most challenging in the Bristol report (Department of Health 2001a) is the statement that 'information should be tailored to the needs, circumstances and wishes of the individual' (Recommendation 5). This approach confirms the movement in law and in the professions towards greater openness and has further ramifications. It implies that nurses have a good knowledge of the patient, perhaps knowing what she or he does and does not want and/or need to know.

The Bristol report suggests that information given to patients should be evidence-based. It should also be presented in different ways, at the appropriate time and with supporting materials designed in partnership with patients. Providing evidence-based information in 'a form comprehensible to patients' (Recommendation 6) requires a high level of competence on the part of the nurse.

This potential movement towards greater transparency has implications for nurses. Are nurses best placed to provide information and answers to questions, and what skills do they require to do so? This clearly depends on the context and on the knowledge and experience of the particular nurse. For example, specialist nurses are likely to have a particularly high level of knowledge and expertise in their own area of practice. As with any other area of practice, the nurse should consider carefully before undertaking an expanded role.

So does Sarah have a right to information in this situation? Clearly, the trend is towards more rather than less disclosure of information in relation to consent. It seems clear that information about the nature of the procedure, including risks and benefits is minimally required. This could be argued for (although it is unlikely that it would need to be) on the basis of Article 8, in particular. As for information about the surgeon's success rates, as health care is becoming increasingly consumerist it seems very possible that, in the future, this information will be freely available and patients/clients can 'shop around' and make more informed choices. It is likely that this will also have resource implications. Nonetheless while the NHS is moving towards greater provision of information the latest guidance falls somewhat short of 'informed consent'. The Department of Health document 'Good Practice in Consent Implementation Guidance' (Department of Health 2001b) states that:

> 'Patients and those close to them will vary in how much information they want; from those who want as much detail as possible, including details of rare risks, to those who ask health professionals to make decisions for them. There will always be an element of clinical judgment in determining what information should be given. However the presumption must be that the patient wishes to be well informed about the risks and benefits of the various options. Where the patient makes it clear (verbally or non-verbally) that they do not wish to be given this level of information, this should be documented.' (p.17)

In the reference guide on consent, regarding examination and treatment, they do little more however than stating the existing legal position stated above although they do note that the General Medical Council has gone further and emphasises that doctors should try to ascertain the needs and priorities of individual patients when giving information regarding treatment options (GMC 1998).

In the case study above, Sarah asks questions. Interestingly the House of Lords in *Sidaway* (1985) indicated that while there was no doctrine of informed consent in English law, patients who ask questions about their treatment should be provided with information in response to their queries. However, subsequently in *Blyth v Bloomsbury Health Authority* (1987) [1993] 4 Med LR 151 (decided in 1987, reported in 1993), the Court of Appeal took the view that a patient – ironically herself a nurse – who had asked questions regarding the risks of Depo Provera was not required to be given full information in response to her queries. Rather it was simply the case that she should be given information in accordance with the approach that a responsible body of professional practice would take in such a situation. In subsequent cases there have been suggestions that a full response should be given where questions have been asked (*Pearce v Bristol NHS Trust* [1999] PIQR P53 CA per Lord Woolf). This is bolstered by Article 8 – the need for respect for autonomy of the individual. Interestingly the Bristol Inquiry Report states that 'patients should be given the opportunity to ask questions' (Recommendation 11). Is the consequence of this that they should be provided with answers? Developments both in the law and in professional practice increasingly suggest that the answer should be yes. The GMC takes this approach and emphasises that where questions are asked they should be answered truthfully (GMC 1998).

It is perhaps somewhat disappointing, in the light of Bristol and the changing attitudes to access to information, that existing Department of Health guidance remains so cautious, particularly in the light of the drivers of the Human Rights Act and Article 8.

The right to refuse consent – adults

Case 3b

> *Molly is seven months pregnant and has been involved in a road traffic accident. She is brought to the Accident and Emergency Department. She has only superficial cuts and complains of abdominal pain. She tells the triage nurse that she believes that she is going into labour and that on no account does she want medical intervention.*

This example poses a number of potential conflicts. Firstly, there may be conflict between the clinical team who want to provide medical interventions and Molly who is opposing them. This may result from a conflict between professionals' perceptions of their duties and patients' rights. Secondly, there is a potential conflict between the interests of the foetus and Molly herself should Molly continue to refuse active therapy. In this case it might be argued that there is a conflict between Molly's right to self-determination and the right of the foetus to life (see Chapter 2 for a further discussion of rights at the beginning of life). The NMC Code of Professional Conduct (2002) states that:

> '3.2 You must respect patients' and clients' autonomy – their right to decide whether or not to undergo any health care intervention – even where a refusal may result in harm or death to themselves or a foetus, unless a court of law orders to the contrary. This right is protected in law although in circumstances where the health of the foetus would be severely compromised by any refusal to give consent, it would be appropriate to discuss this matter fully within the team, and possibly to seek external advice and guidance.'

In relation to the ECHR this example can be seen in terms of Molly's right of self-determination under Article 8. Article 3 may also have relevance, as to compel a patient to receive treatment in such a situation may also be seen in terms of Molly being subjected to inhuman and degrading treatment. This is in accordance with the application of earlier authorities.

Competent patients have the right to refuse medical treatment (*Re J* [1992] 3 WLR 782). The English courts affirmed this principle recently in the high profile case of Ms B, a 43-year-old woman who had become tetraplegic and maintained through artificial ventilation which she requested be removed (*Re B* [2002] 2 All ER 449). Those treating her were of the view that instead she should attend a rehabilitation unit. In authorising the removal of the ventilation in a case which was argued under existing common law provisions rather than under a Human Rights Act basis, Butler Sloss P confirmed the right of the incompetent adult to refuse medical treatment. Moreover she emphasised the importance of involvement of the patient in the decision-making process and that if a dispute arose which is unable to be resolved then other primary care staff should be involved. In this case a small damages award was made of £100 taking account of the fact that she had been treated against her wishes. In a series of cases the English courts were asked to rule on the legality of medical procedures where there was a perceived conflict between maternal decision and foetal rights (*Re S* [1992] 4 All ER 671). Finally, in *Re MB* [1997] 2 FLR 426 the Court of Appeal confirmed that the competent pregnant woman had the right to refuse medical interventions even where the consequence of this would be that the survival of the foetus may be in jeopardy. Butler Sloss LJ commented that:

'A competent woman who has the capacity to decide may, for religious reasons, other reasons, for rational or irrational reasons or for no reason at all, choose not to have medical intervention, even though the consequence may be the death or serious handicap of the child she bears, or her own death. In that event the courts do not have the jurisdiction to declare medical intervention lawful and the question of her own best interests, objectively considered, does not arise.'

Furthermore the Court went on to hold that:

'Although it may seem illogical that a child capable of being born alive is protected by the criminal law from intentional destruction, and by the Abortion Act from termination otherwise than as permitted by the Act, but is not protected from the (irrational) decision of a competent mother not to allow medical intervention to avert the risk of death, this appears to be the present state of the law.'

This approach was followed in *St Georges NHS Trust v S* [1998] 3 All ER 673, which also confirmed that the provisions of the Mental Health Act 1983 could not be used to detain a woman for the purposes of then sanctioning a Caesarean section upon her without her consent. Here Judge LJ held:

'When human life is at stake the pressure to provide an affirmative answer authorising unwarranted medical intervention is very powerful. Nevertheless, the autonomy of each individual requires continuing protection even, perhaps particularly, when the motive for interfering with it is readily understandable and indeed to many would appear commendable.'

These cases have been the subject of considerable academic debate (McHale 2002).

Does the application of the Human Rights Act 1998 now make a difference in such a situation?

One issue is as to whether this situation can be seen in terms of the 'rights' of the foetus at all. At ECHR level the legal status of the foetus is somewhat unclear (this issue is considered further in Chapter 3 below). In *Paton v UK* (1980) 3 EHRR 408 the European Commission of Human Rights held that there was no absolute right to life recognised under Article 2 of the ECHR. The precise scope/application of the Convention regarding the foetus was however left open in this case. In *Open Door Counselling and Dublin Well Woman v Ireland* (1992) 15 EHRR 244 the Commission was asked to rule regarding dissemination of information regarding abortion. One issue which was raised in this case by the Irish Government was that Article 2 safeguarded the rights of the unborn. Interestingly here the Commission indicated that there were situations in which Article 2 could limit the availability of an abortion; however this was not a matter which was further pursued. Furthermore in this case the Court noted that:

> 'National authorities enjoy a wide margin of appreciation in matters of morals, particularly in an area such as the present which touches on matters of belief concerning the nature of human life.'

Havers and Sheldon have commented that 'Just as the margin of appreciation doctrine appears to have restricted the courts in this particular sensitive moral question, so might domestic courts be persuaded that any development of the law in this area is a matter best left to Parliament'.

So does Molly have a right to refuse treatment? It seems that, given the lack of clarity in relation to the legal status of the foetus and increasing acceptance of patient autonomy, at present her refusal should be upheld. Some guidance was set out in *St Georges Hospital NHS Trust v S* [1998] 3 All ER 673 which provides that in such cases where there are concerns regarding capacity the issue should be referred to the courts for determination.

Right to refuse treatment – children

Case 3c

Joseph is 17 years old and has been chronically ill with leukaemia for two years. His parents have been told that his best chance of survival is to have a bone marrow transplant. The family belongs to a religious group which opposes aggressive medical interventions. In speaking with doctors, Joseph states that he wants no further treatment and that 'God should decide' whether he lives or dies. Linda is Joseph's named nurse and finds his decision difficult.

In this type of situation, questions arise about the child's competence. The child patient poses difficulties in determining the boundaries of consent to treatment.

Under current English law children over the age of 16 have the right under Section 8 of the Family Law Reform Act 1969 to consent to surgical, medical and dental treatment. Children under the age of 16 may still have competence to consent to treatment if they have 'sufficient maturity' to do so (*Gillick v West Norfolk and Wisbech AHA* [1985] 3 All ER 402). The determination of whether they do have such maturity is a decision-relative test and thus varies from situation to situation. An adolescent may have the maturity to make decisions regarding one clinical procedure while not having the maturity to determine another.

That does not mean that they have an unfettered right in the consent process even if they are over 16. First, the 1969 Act does not apply in certain situations – for example, it does not apply to blood and organ donation (*Re W* [1992] 4 All ER 627). Second, the provisions regarding consent do not apply equally in the context of refusal of treatment. The Court of Appeal has confirmed that in a situation in which even a competent adolescent refuses treatment, consent may be given either by the person with parental responsibility or by the court (*Re R* [1991] 4 All ER 177 and *Re W* [1992] 4 All ER 627). This would suggest that in such a situation even where he refuses treatment this refusal is unlikely to be respected by the courts. In *Re M* [1999] 2 FLR 1097 a 15-year-old girl refused a heart transplant. She was unhappy not only with the period of post-operative therapy but also with the notion that she would be carrying the heart of another person around inside her. Johnson J however held that she was incompetent and that she had not been able to come to terms with the situation which faced her. Moreover, any consequent risks of the operation were outweighed by the fact that she would otherwise die without the transplant.

Garwood-Gowers (2001) suggests that there are three reasons which could be advanced for treating competent minors different from their adult counterparts. Firstly that children are different *per se*. However he suggests that while teenagers have more limited understanding of such things as risk levels he notes that this is offset by the fact that the law does require different levels of understanding in the determination of competency which is a decision-relative test. Secondly, there is the argument that medical professionals need legal safeguards in relation to such decisions, but he refutes this on the basis that similar protections are not given regarding decision making in relation to adults. Thirdly, it might be argued that there are practical difficulties regarding competency – but as he notes, this is an issue which is undertaken already regarding adults.

Will the HRA will make a difference in such cases? A number of Convention rights are potentially, at least, applicable. Article 3, for example – the prohibition on torture and degrading treatment – forcing a protesting minor perhaps through physical restraint to undergo unwanted therapy may fall within this category. However the European Court of Human Rights has interpreted this provision somewhat restrictively in the context of medical treatment. Where a measure is regarded as being therapeutically necessary then this will not be regarded as being inhuman and degrading (*Herczegfalvy v Austria* (Series A, No 242- B(1992)).

Secondly, could enforcing treatment here also be regarded as a violation of Article 5 – the right to liberty and security of the person? Garwood-Gowers (2001) has commented that it is clear from ECHR caselaw that liberty and security here can be regarded 'in a unitary fashion'. However in the past in a number of cases in which the adolescent has objected to therapy but a parent has approved of the therapy going ahead then the Court has sanctioned the treatment. In *Nielson v Denmark* (Report 12 March 1987, Series A, No 144) a complaint was made by a person who had been hospitalised in a psychiatric hospital at the age of 12 against his will but with his mother's acquiescence. Here the European Court of Human Rights found that there was no violation of the Convention. It was held that Article 5 was inapplicable as the power of the parent to make decisions on behalf of the child applied in such a case and that here 'he was still of an age where it would be normal for the decision to be made by the parent even against the wishes of the child'. Garwood-Gowers (2001) speculates as to whether the English courts will be prepared to take a different approach to this particular issue. Certainly as he notes there is an issue in this case as to whether the boy was competent to make the decision. It may be the case, as he comments, that:

> 'the Court might if faced with a competent minor decide that there is either a general right of self-determination or one that exists in all but exceptional circumstances such as where forced intervention is necessary as a life saving measure or at least to avert a prospectively grave impact on health.' (Garwood-Gowers 2001, p.237)

Thirdly, Article 8, the infringement of personal autonomy, may also be applicable. As was stated in *X v Austria* (App No 8278/78 (1979) 18 D&R 154, a requirement to take a blood test was found to be in breach of the ECHR. Here it was stated that:

> 'A compulsory medical intervention, even if it is of minor importance, must be considered as an interference with this right.' (p.156)

This approach has also been confirmed in *Re A (children)(conjoined twins medical treatment)* [2001] FLR 1 where Brooke LJ confirmed that Article 8(1) can be interpreted as a right not to be subjected to compulsory medical intervention. Nonetheless Article 8 is a qualified right and thus subject to a series of other 'public interest' considerations.

Fourthly, Article 9 may be applicable where the treatment refusal is connected to a religious/cultural belief. Here the refusal of treatment is on the grounds of a belief. In the past however the courts have been unsympathetic to such claims. In *Re A (conjoined twins)* [2001] 1 FLR 1, parental opposition to surgery to separate conjoined twins on religious grounds (they were Roman Catholics) was overborne. In *Re L (medical treatment)* [1998] 2 FLR 810, L, a Jehovah's Witness, was 14 years of age. She had suffered severe scalds having fallen into a bath of hot water. 54% of her body surface had severe burns and 40% had third degree burns. Surgery and a blood transfusion were required. She verbally refused the blood transfusion and she was also carrying a

Jehovah's Witness card. Sir Stephen Brown held that in this case she was not 'Gillick competent'. (One factor in this case was that she had not been informed by her family of the full nature of her condition.)

Finally an option considered by Garwood-Gowers is that of the application of Article 14 – the prohibition on discrimination when read in conjunction with Articles 5 and 8.

> 'In using Article 14 in conjunction with Article 5 it can be said that denying competent minors the legal right to self-determination with respect to medical intervention discriminates against them in terms of liberty and security.' (Garwood-Gowers 2001, p.240)

An alternative approach is to argue that where the child is not competent to make the decision themselves, a decision to authorise treatment in the face of objection from both child and parent has the effect that it infringes the mother's rights under the Convention, such as Article 8(1) and Article 9 (Michalowski 2001).

In the past parental objections to clinical procedures being undertaken have generally been overridden by the courts. There is one notable exception, that of *Re T* [1997] 1 WLR 242 where a parental decision not to go ahead with a liver transplant was upheld even though in this case very high success rates were suggested – of up to 90% in some reports (Fox & McHale 1997). The judgment in this case noted the close bond between mother and child and the fact that she would have to care for the child. Butler Sloss LJ stated that:

> 'The welfare of the child is the paramount consideration and I recognise the 'very strong presumption in favour of a course of action which will prolong life' and the inevitable consequences for the child of not giving consent. But to prolong life... is not the sole objective of the court and to require it at the expense of other considerations may not be in a child's best interests. The prospect of forcing the devoted mother of this young baby to the consequences of this major invasive surgery lead me to the conclusion... that it is not in the best interests of this child to give consent... I believe that the best interests of the child require that his future treatment should be left in the hands of his devoted parents.'

Michaelowski (2001) considers the extent to which this decision would be upheld in the light of the ECHR and rights such as Articles 2 and Articles 3. She comments that a case such as this one, involving a risky invasive procedure which may if unsuccessful have shortened the life of the child, will involve a careful risk assessment being undertaken by the courts.

However while the parental human rights may be argued equally they may be subject to limitations. Articles 8 and 9 as noted above are 'qualified' rights. In a case concerning access by a mother to her child *Johansen v Norway* (1996) 23 EHRR 33 it was held by the European Court of Human Rights that in determining the balancing test required under Article 8:

> 'The Court will attach particular importance to the best interests of the child, which, depending on their nature and seriousness, may override

those of the parents. In particular... the parent cannot be entitled under Art 8 of the Convention to have such measures taken as would harm the child's health and development.'

Michalowski has suggested that:

'Applied to treatment decisions on behalf of young children, this decision seems to suggest that, on balance, the parental right will be outweighed where the treatment decision was found to impair the child's health. Consequently, parental claims of a violation of their right under Art 8 will rarely be successful in this context.' (Michalowski 2001 p.246)

Nonetheless, as she comments, certain cases indicate that there is a right for the parents to be consulted regarding the proposed medical intervention and to be involved in the decision making process (e.g. *R v UK* Series A No 121-C (1987) paras 68 and 69).

How the courts will proceed in the light of the Human Rights Act is uncertain. It is suggested that in the case of very young children it is likely that judicial approaches will be cautious and may militate in favour of adherence to professional judgment. More questionable is the application of the 1998 Act in a case, as here, of an older child. Situations such as that of Joseph above present particular challenges for nurses. On the one hand, they may acknowledge a professional obligation to advocate on behalf of the child but, on the other, they may find it difficult to accept the child's stated wish to die. A graphic illustration of the consequences which may ensue if treatment is compelled is provided by *Re E (a minor)(wardship: medical treatment)* [1993] 1 FLR 386. Here Ward J held that the minor did not understand the full implications of the consequences of his decision. Moreover he went onto say that:

'I respect this boy's profession of faith but I cannot discount at least the possibility that he may in later years suffer some diminution in his convictions. There is no settled certainty about matters of this kind.'

However, when the boy reached 18 he refused any further treatment and then died.

It may be that the courts may, in the future, be more willing to take a different approach.

Rights, consent and the incompetent adult patient

Case 3d

> *Samantha is twenty years old and lives in a community home for those with learning disabilities. She has recently developed a relationship with another client. Her mother shares her concern that her daughter may become pregnant. She tells staff that she wants Samantha sterilised.*

Samantha is 20 and is considered an adult in law. An important issue which arises here is the application of human rights principles. Article 8 may be applicable and this may also be considered along with Article 12, the right to marry and found a family. Sterilisation can be seen as an attack upon these rights. Initially there was judicial reference to reproductive rights. In *Re D* [1976] All ER 326, Heilbron J, in refusing to authorise a non-therapeutic sterilisation operation upon an 11-year-old child with Sotos syndrome stated that:

'The type of operation proposed is one which involves the deprivation of a basic human right, namely the right of a woman to reproduce, and therefore would, if performed on a woman for non-therapeutic reasons and without her consent, be a violation of such a right.'

However subsequently the courts did not effectively engage with the rights of the mentally incompetent. Indeed in *Re B* [1987] 2 All ER 206 which concerned the decision to sterilise a mentally handicapped girl of 17 Lord Hailsham stated that:

'To talk of the basic right to reproduce of an individual who... is unable to form any maternal instincts or to care for a child, appears to me wholly to part company with reality.'

Earlier decisions emphasised the respect given to medical judgment. In the case of the mentally incompetent adult no one has the right to make treatment decisions on their behalf. This was confirmed by the House of Lords in *Re F* in 1990. Instead treatment may be given under the doctrine of necessity where it is in the best interests of the patient. Traditionally the determination of best interests in such a situation was referable to a responsible body of medical opinion (*Bolam v Friern Hospital Management Committee* [1957] 2 All ER 188). However, recently the courts have shown that they are prepared to take a broader approach. In *Re SL* [2000] 3 WLR 1288 the courts undertook a broader approach to best interests referable to the social and ethical context within which the decision was being made. Thorpe J held that:

'In practice the dispute will generally require the court to choose between two or more possible treatments both or all of which comfortably pass the *Bolam* test. As most of us know from experience a patient contemplating treatment for a physical condition or illness is often offered a range of alternatives with counter-balancing advantages and disadvantages. One of the most important services provided by a consultant is to explain the available alternatives to the patient. Particularly concentrating on those features of advantages and disadvantage most relevant to his needs and circumstances. In a developing relationship of confidence the consultant then guides the patient to make the choice that best suits his circumstances and personality. It is precisely because the patient is prevented by disability from that exchange that the judge must in certain circumstances either exercise the choice between alternative available treatments or perhaps refuse any form of treatment. In deciding what is best for the disabled patient the judge must have regard to the patient's welfare as the paramount consideration. That embraces issues far wider than the medical. Indeed it would be undesirable and probably impossible to set bounds to what is relevant to a welfare determination.'

In this case the mother of S, a 28-year-old woman with severe learning disabilities, sought a declaration that it would be in S's best interests to undergo sterilisation and/or hysterectomy. Initially it was ruled that the declaration be granted and that hysterectomy was the most appropriate solution. The Official Solicitor appealed against the declaration and it was held that the judge had erred as the expert evidence had been unanimously in favour of intrauterine contraception as a less invasive procedure. Thus, it was held that the correct decision was that the insertion of the intrauterine device was in the best interests of S as it was the least invasive option and was not irreversible.

Where it is sought to sterilise a patient guidance in a Practice Note ([2001] 2 FLR 158) provides that applications should be made to the Family Division of the High Court, usually by the Official Solicitor with the patient being represented. Evidence is required normally as to the existing capacity of the patient and also regarding the future capacity of the patient to take decisions. If they lack capacity evidence will be sought as to probability of conception/damage which is expected to result from menstruation/conception, medical/surgical techniques which are available and any less restrictive alternatives.

How then will human rights considerations apply in this context? As Wicks (2001) notes, the right under Article 12 is far from absolute in nature and the limitations include the fact that the right may only be exercised in relation to national laws which govern the right. It was noted in *Rees v UK* (1986) (Series A No 106 para 50) that the qualifications to Article 12 'must not restrict or reduce the right in such a way or to such an extent that the very essence of the right is impaired'. Wicks suggests that the existing law cannot be seen as a violation of the right (Wicks 2001 at page 36).

There has only been limited judicial discussion of the application of the ECHR in relation to such cases following the Human Rights Act 1998. *Re A (medical treatment: male sterilisation)* [2000] FLR 193, a case decided prior to the enactment of the 1998 Act, concerned sterilisation of a 28-year-old man with Down's Syndrome assessed as borderline between significant and severe intelligence impairment. He was sexually aware and active but was unable to make a decision himself regarding the sterilisation. His mother supported his sterilisation. The Court of Appeal held that the sterilisation should not at present go ahead. Dame Elisabeth Butler Sloss P indicated that at a time when there was soon to be direct application of the European Convention of Human Rights in English law the court should be slow to take a step which may infringe the rights of those who are unable to act for themselves. The Court of Appeal emphasised that the patient's best interests was something which was different from the interests of carers or others. They did indicate that the carers' interests may be a relevant consideration to take into account.

Wicks (2001) has commented that whilst in practice establishing breach of the ECHR in this situation is thus unlikely, this does not mean that they are not raising issues of serious concern.

'The right of a mentally handicapped woman to found a family is just as important as any other woman's right to do so. Indeed it may be even more vital to acknowledge and protect her right because it is more likely to be threatened.' (ibid)

Rights and advance directives

Case 3e

> *Jill collapsed at home, sustaining a head injury which bled profusely, and was taken unconscious to the Accident and Emergency Department. She requires treatment as she has lost blood. In searching for identification, the staff nurse finds that Jill is in possession of an advance directive which states that she does not wish to have a blood transfusion.*

However, what of the situation as here, where a person temporarily lacks capacity? The right to refuse treatment can be seen as potentially at least supported by Article 3, Article 8, the right to privacy, and Article 9, the respect given to freedom of conscience and religion. The law allows treatment to be given in an emergency situation on the basis of common law 'necessity'. In such a situation, though, 'necessity' refers to undertaking those procedures which are immediately necessary and no more. There is a further issue here which is that of the advance directive. In the UK (in contrast to the USA) there is no legislation governing this issue; however, although there were proposals made by the Law Commission in their 1995 report on Mental Incapacity for the introduction of legislation on this issue this was not taken up by the Government (LCD 1997; LCD 1999). Nonetheless, a competent adult's right to make treatment decisions does include both the right to consent and to refuse that treatment (*Re T* [1992]). This includes both oral and written refusals. In a well-known Canadian case *Malette v Shulman* (1987) 47 DLR 18, a Jehovah's Witness carried a card refusing blood transfusion. Nonethless, a transfusion was administered. The doctor had doubts as to the applicability of the card in that specific case. However the patient subsequently succeeded in an action for damages. Donnelly J held:

'That message is unqualified. It does not exempt life-threatening perils. On the face of the card, its message is seen to be rooted in religious conviction. Its obvious purpose as a card is as protection, to speak in circumstances when the card carrier cannot.'

The claimant succeeded in an action for battery. One interesting question is whether the impact of the refusal is strengthened where this is refusal based on conscience or belief through the application of Article 9, or weakened through concerns to safeguard the sanctity of life under Article 2. In *Malette v Shulman* Donnelly stated that:

> 'However sacred life may be, fair social comment admits that certain aspects of life are properly held to be more important than life itself. Such proud and honourable motivations are long entrenched in society whether it be patriotism in war, duty by law enforcement officers, protection of the life of a spouse, son or daughter, death before dishonour, death before loss of liberty or religious martyrdom. Refusal of medical treatment on religious grounds is such a value.' (p.47)

Wicks (2001) comments that sanctity of life as a principle can also be seen as being something which is ultimately based upon religion. She argues:

> 'Religion can compel a patient to refuse treatment, it can equally compel a doctor to impose treatment without consent. In a society in which different religions, different beliefs and different interpretations of those religions and beliefs co-exist it is the requirement of the patient's religion, as interpreted by the patient, which must be upheld. No less significantly however the other secular beliefs and wishes of the patient should also be upheld. This is the consequence of the right to self-determination.'

The English courts now seem to be following this example and certainly in the case of patients who choose to have life-saving treatment withdrawn, such as that of Miss B, they have taken this approach. We return to this issue in Chapter 8 below.

Conclusion

Changes are apparent in health care in relation to consent. There is a movement towards an enhanced provision of information to patients particularly in the light of the Bristol Inquiry Report (Kennedy et al 2001). At the same time there has been enhanced judicial scrutiny of professional practice. In contrast, in relation to issues of capacity and overriding the choice of the patient (whether child or adult), the situation is considerably different. It remains to be seen as to whether in this area the courts are willing to take a different approach driven by concern to safeguard the patient's human rights. While in the past there was much use of the rhetoric of respect for rights such as autonomy, the reality has been somewhat different. It is to be hoped that there is an increasing judicial realisation of the nature/importance of respect for the human rights of the individual patient.

REFERENCES

Department of Health 2001a Learning from Bristol: The Department of Health's response to the report of the public inquiry into children's heart surgery at Bristol Royal Infirmary 1984-1995. Cm 5363: 139-140

Department of Health 2001b Reference guide to consent for examination or treatment. http://www.doh.gov.uk/consent

Fox M, McHale J 1997 In whose best interests? Modern Law Review 60: 700

Garwood-Gowers A 2001 Time for competent minors to have the same right of self-determination as competent adults with respect to medical intervention. In: Garwood-Gowers A, Tingle J Healthcare law: The impact of the Human Rights Act 1998. Cavendish, London

General Medical Council 1998 Seeking patients' consent: The ethical considerations. GMC, London

Havers P, Sheldon N The impact of the convention in medical law. In: Havers P (ed) (ed) An introduction to himan rights and the common law. Oxford University Press, Oxford

Lord Chancellor's Department 1997 Who decides? LCD, London

Lord Chancellor's Department 1999 Making decisions. LCD, London

McHale J 2002 Consent and the competent adult patient. In: Tingle J, Cribb A (eds) Nursing law and ethics, 2nd edn. Blackwell Scientific, Oxford

Michalowski S 2001 Young children, best interests and the Human Rights Act 1998. In: Garwood-Gowers A, Tingle J Healthcare law: The impact of the Human Rights Act 1998. Cavendish, London

NMC 2002 Code of professional conduct. Nursing & Midwifery Council, London

Wicks E 2001 The right to refuse medical treatment under the European Convention of Human Rights. Medical Law Review 9: 17

Chapter 4

Human rights and mental health care

Introduction

It is estimated that, at any one time, approximately one in six people of working age will have a mental health problem such as anxiety or depression. Psychotic illness will affect one person in 250 (NHS 1999). It is not only nurses who work in designated mental health areas who need to consider the significance of mental health (UKCC 2000) and associated rights issues. School nurses have to respond to sometimes serious mental health problems in children and adolescents; midwives and health visitors have to respond to women who suffer from postnatal depression, self-harm and other mental health problems; and all nurses, whether in hospital or in the community, require an understanding of the needs and rights of those with mental health problems and also need to consider the importance of mental health promotion. Standard 1 of the National Service Framework for Mental Health (NHS 1999) states:

'Health and social services should:

- promote mental health for all, working with individuals and communities

- combat discrimination against individuals and groups with mental health problems, and promote their social inclusion.'

Mental health work poses some of the most challenging rights issues. It is often the case that in the pursuit of the well-being of the individual and the safety and security of the family and society at large, the rights of the individual will be curtailed. Those with mental health problems are also liable to be misunderstood and their illness stigmatised.

The UKCC (now the Nursing and Midwifery Council) acknowledged the special nature of mental health and learning disabilities nursing in publishing specific guidelines in 1998, discussing issues such as accountability, consent, autonomy, confidentiality, risk management and advocacy (UKCC 1998). Advocacy is particularly challenging in mental health practice as nurses who provide care, act as advocates and promote self-advocacy may also, at times, be involved in sectioning patients under the Mental Health Act 1983, thus depriving them of their freedom. The UKCC (1998) acknowledged these challenges and pointed out that 'in most instances, an independent advocate can provide more objective support to clients' (Section 30, p.14). The Department of Health has recently issued recommendations for good practice in relation to independent specialist advocacy for those who are 'subject to the powers of mental health legislation in England and Wales'. One of the purposes of specialist advocacy is:

'to help safeguard the rights of service users – both rights under mental health policy and law, and rights as citizens.' (http://www.doh.gov.uk/ mentalhealth/advocacy/summary.htm)

The Code of Professional Conduct (NMC 2002) directs nurses in mental health care, as in other areas of practice, to respect clients, obtain consent, maintain confidentiality, co-operate with team members (including the client and family), maintain professional knowledge and competence, be trustworthy and minimise risk.

As with other areas of health care practice, it is impossible to predict which articles will be appealed to in future mental health rights challenges but it seems plausible that Article 2 (right to life), Article 3 (prohibition of torture, inhuman and degrading treatment), Article 4 (right to liberty and security), Article 6 (right to a fair trial), Article 8 (right to respect for private and family life), Article 9 (freedom of thought, conscience and religion), Article 10 (freedom of expression) and Article 14 (prohibition of discrimination) will have particular relevance.

In this chapter, we will provide some background discussion regarding mental health legislation, including an overview of the proposed new Mental Health Act. We will then explore the following issues: the right to treatment and the right to refuse treatment; the right to a therapeutic environment; rights to liberty and security. Some issues concerning mental health and privacy are discussed in Chapter 5.

The 1999 edition of the Code of Practice relating to the Mental Health Act 1983 emphasises the importance of rights. The first broad principle states that people to whom the Act applies should:

'receive recognition of their basic rights under the European Convention on Human Rights (ECHR).'

The 1998 Human Rights Act now incorporates the Convention and its jurisprudence into English law. This framework applies to all patients in the mental health care system, not only those detained under the Mental Health Act. In thinking about the implications of the HRA 1998 on mental health practice, we need to consider what mental health and illness involves and what the relationship is between mental health and human rights.

In Chapter 1 we discussed the uncertain definitional territory of health. Definitions of mental health and mental illness are particularly challenging. As with health generally, positive and negative definitions of mental health have been suggested. A negative view of mental health focuses on the absence of disease and illness. Disease relates to the objective existence, and detection, of some abnormality or pathology. While some mental health problems lend themselves to such an explanation (for example, organic conditions such as Alzheimer's disease), most do not. Illness is a subjective term and relates to the individual's subjective experience of loss of health, generally described in terms of symptoms or function loss. Subjective reports of illness are not always reliable indicators of the mental health status of individuals. There may be a difference of opinion between the patient/client and professionals as to the former's mental health/illness status.

It has been pointed out that defining mental illness is a matter of fact and value. These positions allow for the role of science in psychiatry while also recognising that values have a significant role in treatment choice and diagnosis (see Fulford in Chadwick 1998). Positive definitions of mental health have suggested that mental well-being can be related to pleasure or to autonomy (see Coombes in Chadwick 1998).

The lack of a definition of mental illness in the 1983 Mental Health Act is telling. Defining mental illness is undoubtedly challenging and generally it is given meaning in the specification of a list of particular illnesses with associated characteristics. Section 1(2) of the 1983 Act instead defines 'mental disorder' under this section as 'mental illness, arrested or incomplete development of mind, psychopathic disorder and any other disability of mind'. The Act does not define mental illness but it should be given its ordinary meaning (*W v L* [1974] QB 711). This definition expressly excludes sexual deviations and alcoholism (Section 1(3) Mental Health Act 1983). Psychopathic disorder is defined as being a disorder/disability of mind (whether or not including significant impairment of intelligence) resulting in abnormally aggressive or seriously irresponsible conduct.

Historically, there is evidence that the mental health 'care' system itself promoted dependence and, in the process of institutionalisation (see, for example, Goffman 1961) denied individuals the opportunity to make decisions for themselves.

The relationships discussed in Chapter 1 relating to health and human rights generally also have application to mental health (Mann et al 1999, Chapter 1). First, health policies and practices have the potential to impact, positively or negatively, on human rights. Mental health policy permits the exercise of government power both to promote the welfare of the individual, the family and society and also to deprive individuals of their right to liberty, privacy and property. Secondly, rights violations such as torture, abuse, neglect and violations of privacy can have a detrimental impact on health, particularly mental health. Finally, the positive promotion of human rights and mental health are 'inextricably linked' in that they are both concerned with the well-being of human beings.

As discussed in Chapter 1, it is not the case that individuals have a right to all that might make them healthy. This also applies to mental health. There are many factors which have the potential to contribute to mental health which are beyond the remit of the mental health services. So what rights do users of the mental health services and their families have?

In addition to the HRA 1998, a number of other very significant rights frameworks are relevant to mental health practice. The United Nations Charter (1945), for example, requires member states to promote universal respect for the human rights of all, regardless of individual differences. There has already been discussion in Chapter 1 of the right to health as outlined in the Universal Declaration of Human Rights (1948) and in the International Covenants on Human Rights which also have relevance to mental health practice. The International Covenant on Civil and Political Rights (ICCPR 1966, ratified 1976), for example, emphasises fundamental and absolute rights such as the right to life (Article 6), freedom from torture, cruel and inhuman treatment (Article 7) and the right to recognition as a person before the law (Article 16). The International Covenant on Economic, Social and Cultural Rights (ICESCR 1966, ratified 1976) makes explicit positive rights which include family protection, an adequate standard of living and education. Article 12 states 'the right of everyone to the highest standard of physical and mental health' (Gostin 2000). Towards the end of the 'Decade for Disabled Persons' (1983-1992), the General Assembly of the United Nations adopted 'Principles of the Protection of Persons with Mental Illness and for the Improvement of Mental Health Care (MI Principles 1991 see http://www.un.org/ documents/ga/res/46/ a46r119.htm). There are 25 principles in all and they outline the fundamental rights and basic freedoms to which those with mental health problems are entitled (Principle 1). They also cover more specific areas such as the protection of minors (Principle 2), the right to live in the community (Principle 3), the right to have appropriate diagnosis, examination, care and treatment (Principles 4, 5, 7, 8 and 9), the right to confidentiality (Principle 6), and the right to consent (Principle 11). It is emphasised that 'every effort should be made to avoid involuntary admissions' (Principle 15) and that where an involuntary admission is necessary there is a review process and appropriate safeguards in place (Principles 16, 17 and 18). The right to make a complaint and to ensure that there are appropriate inspection and investigation processes are also included (Principles 22 and 23). Although United Nations Assembly resolutions are not 'directly binding' on states they do have practical significance in their establishment of normative principles and standards.

There has been and continues to be much concern about the vulnerability and treatment of clients/patients in mental 'health' institutions and in the community. Globally, there was optimism that, with the collapse of the Soviet Union, the abuse of psychiatry would decrease. There is, however, current concern about alleged inappropriate psychiatric hospitalisation of dissidents in the People's Republic of China. The concept of 'political psychosis' has been discussed by a number of researchers (Freedman 2001).

There has also been concern expressed about the involvement of health care professionals in human rights violations such as in relation to capital punishment – psychiatrists who, for example, treat a psychotic inmate on 'death row' to make him competent for execution. Freedman (2001) writes of the 'novel rationale' said to justify departure from medical ethical codes which holds that 'when a psychiatrist acts in a criminal justice case, that individual is no longer a psychiatrist and is not bound by psychiatric ethics'.

Fortunately, nurses and doctors in Britain do not have to contend with the challenges of capital punishment, but they do have to consider how to respond to violations of rights in mental health institutions and in relation to, for example, those in prison who have mental health problems. There is no room for complacency. A BMA report (BMA 1992) highlighted 'systematic failures' in relation to the care of those with mental illness and learning disabilities in Europe. In 1996, a patient in the Personality Disorder Unit at Ashworth Special Hospital made a number of serious accusations about drug and alcohol misuse, paedophile activity and pornography, and financial irregularities. It was revealed that earlier complaints had not been investigated or passed on to the Department of Health (BMA 2001). A number of cases in the last two decades have also highlighted rights violations of a particularly vulnerable group – older people with mental health problems. Sadly, nurses were implicated in these. In March 2000, for example, it was reported that elderly patients in Carlisle were subject to 'degrading and cruel treatment' by nurses (BMA 2001 p.294).

Major developments have taken place in mental health services and policy in the United Kingdom. There has been a movement from in-patient services to community care, and there have been reviews of mental health legislation. There have also been policy discussions on issues such as capacity and incapacity (see, for example, 'Making Decisions' 1999). The introduction of the National Service Framework for mental health (September 1999) is also a significant development with the stated aims of 'driv[ing] up quality and remov[ing] the wide and unacceptable variations in provision' (p.5).

The provision of mental health care and powers of treatment and detention are primarily regulated under the Mental Health Act 1983 (see further Gostin 2000; Bartlett & Sandland 2000). This legislation enables patients to be detained firstly for assessment for a period of up to 28 days (Section 2) and then for treatment for an initial period of up to six months, which may then be renewed (Section 3). There are also emergency powers of detention for up to 72 hours (Section 4) and specific powers given to police officers under Section 136). The rights and interests of patients detained under the legislation are safeguarded through the operation of the Mental Health Act Commission, a body which is also responsible for the development of the Mental Health Act Code of Practice. It has powers to investigate care provided to patients held under the Act. The Act enables treatment to be given on a compulsory basis in hospitals. Care may also be given to patients in the community, although the legislation in this area does not sanction compulsion in therapy (Mental Health (Patients in the Community) Act 1995). There are also a series of powers relating to detention of persons who have been involved in the criminal justice system. (For further discussion on this issue see Laing; Glover-Thomas 2002.)

The most significant legal development relating to human rights and mental health law is likely to be the new Mental Health Act proposed in the Department of Health White Paper and Draft Bill (Department of Health 2000; 2002). A consultation process is currently underway. This major reform of the mental health system began in 1998 with the appointment by the government of an Expert Group with Professor Genevra Richardson as chair (Department of Health 1999a). Its brief was to consider the prospects for reform in the area, and this led to a Green Paper (Department of Health 1999b), a White Paper (Department of Health 2000) and a draft Bill produced in Summer 2002 (Department of Health 2002). The Government's proposals differ considerably from the initial reform proposals advocated by Richardson which were rooted in a rights base (Richardson 1999). The publication of the draft Bill led to a storm of protest. Nonetheless, it appears that the Government intends to press ahead with it.

The Mental Health Act reforms propose replacing the existing admissions structure with a single admission for assessment for 28 days. All further assessments would be subject to approval by a Mental Health Tribunal. The emphasis in the Richardson report upon the need for capacity has been abandoned. The current emphasis placed upon treatability in the Mental Health Act 1983 has been rejected and, controversially, the proposals sanction detention on the basis of risk where there is no prospect of further treatment. The extent to which these proposals conform with the Human Rights Act on this issue may be questioned. Interestingly, in October 2001, a Scottish case, *Anderson v Scottish Ministers* [2002] 3 WLR 1460 considered a provision of the Mental Health (Public Safety and Appeals) (Scotland) Act 1999 which enabled an appeal for detention from a restriction order not to be granted where the patient was suffering from a mental disorder such that it was necessary to protect the public for the person to be continued to be detained in hospital, whether or not this was for medical treatment. This was upheld as not being incompatible with Article 5 of the ECHR. This case is of particular significance in that it legitimated the continued detention of untreatable psychopaths (Fennell 2002). The Draft Bill also controversially contains proposals for the first time to enable compulsory treatment in the community. New provisions regarding the treatment of children are to be introduced which in particular recognise the need for children (particularly older children) to have a greater say in their treatment decisions. Where children oppose therapy, parental authority will apply for a 28-day period, after which treatment must be authorised by a Mental Health Tribunal.

These proposals are being introduced in the light of the application of Articles 5 and 8 of the ECHR. It is also proposed that the Mental Health Act Commission will be replaced, and powers to scrutinise and inspect will be given to the new health care inspectorate which the Government has already created. While the proposals have received almost universal condemnation the Government still appears committed to them.

Right to treatment and to refuse treatment for mental disorder

Case 4a

> *Jack is 59, and has been admitted voluntarily to an acute psychiatric ward. In discussion with his key nurse, Jack says that he feels very low and that he has nothing to live for. In the course of a risk assessment he reveals that, at times, he feels like taking his own life. He says that he would like to be helped but that he does not want to take anti-depressants, as recommended by the team, or to have electro-convulsive therapy (ECT) as on an earlier admission.*

Clients like Jack, who receive mental health services, sometimes are at risk of self-harm or suicide and occasionally pose a threat to the lives of others. Recent cases such as *Osman v United Kingdom* [2000] 29 EHRR 245 indicate a positive obligation to protect life. It has been suggested that an actual or attempted suicide could give rise to a breach of Article 2 (right to life) and also that more 'robust safeguards' will have to be put in place regarding risk assessment and management, level of observation and staffing levels and prescribing policies (Persaud & Hewitt 2001).

One of the most significant standard-setting frameworks is the National Service Framework (NHS 1999) and it is hoped that this will make a significant contribution to creating and supporting therapeutic environments. Standard 7, for example, refers to the prevention of suicide and would have relevance to the case of Jack above.

The basic principles of consent to treatment at common law as discussed in Chapter 3 are as applicable to psychiatric patients as to those with a physical illness. This is emphasised in the NMC Code (2002 p.5) as follows:

> '3.7 The principles of obtaining consent apply equally to those people who have a mental illness.'

However this vignette also raises questions of consent and refusal of treatment. Specific consent issues have been dealt with in the previous chapter, and the relevance of capacity or competence to consent discussed. In this case, Jack is entitled to information about treatment options, and professionals should explore the client's understanding of, and views about, the treatments offered and the treatments available. It needs also to be said that there continues to be uncertainty about 'best practice' in psychiatry and much controversy about treatments such as electro-convulsive therapy. In the future there will be guidance here from the National Institute for Clinical Excellence (NICE). The Institute is currently working on clinical guidelines in relation to the management of depression (see http://www.nice.org.uk), due for issue in September 2003, and the Institute is also undertaking a technology appraisal of ECT (http://www.nice.org.uk), due for issue in December 2002. The ECT review has been welcomed by professionals and service users (Batty 2001). As a voluntary patient, Jack has a right to refuse treatment. His right to refuse may be curtailed should he be sectioned under the Mental Health Act 1983 in the event of a deterioration in his condition, and treatment may be deemed necessary.

Although the Human Rights Act does not explicitly address issues of consent, it can be argued that imposing treatment without consent violates Article 3, the right not to be subjected to torture and inhuman/degrading treatment. However where a procedure is a therapeutic necessity then it is not considered to be inhuman/degrading treatment (*Herczegfalvy v Austria* (1992) 15 EHRR 437).

As discussed above, the United Nations General Assembly 'Principles for the Protection of Persons with Mental Illness and the Improvement of Mental Health Care' emphasises consent to treatment (Principle 11). The general limitation clause to these principles states:

> 'The exercise of the rights set forth in the present Principles may be subject only to such limitations as are prescribed by law and are necessary to protect the health or safety of the person concerned or of others, or otherwise to protect public safety, order, health or morals or the fundamental rights and freedoms of others.' (General Assembly UN 1991)

Under Part IV of the Mental Health Act 1983 some treatments may be given, in some circumstances, without the consent of the patient. 'Treatment' includes medication and nursing care but may also extend to, for instance, feeding, if the patient's mental illness leads to the refusal of food (*B v Croyden HA* [1995] 1 All ER 683); *Riverside Mental Health Trust v Fox* [1994] 2 Med Law Review 95). The power extends for a three month period. Psychosurgery and other procedures (governed by regulations) including the surgical implantation of hormones are regulated under Section 57. The administration of medicines and electro-convulsive therapy (ECT) are governed by Section 58 of the 1983 Act. Special authorisation under this Section is needed regarding medicines once three months have passed from the point when the patient was first admitted and given treatment for his or her mental disorder. Section 58 provides that either the patient must consent or, where they refuse, a second opinion approved doctor may authorise treatment.

The doctor must state that either the patient is not competent because he or she cannot understand the nature, purpose or likely effects of treatment or that, while the patient is competent and is refusing treatment, in view of the likelihood of it alleviating or preventing a deterioration in the patient's condition treatment should be given (S.58(3)(b)). In reaching this conclusion the second opinion approved doctor should also consult two other persons professionally involved in that person's care. At least one of these persons is a nurse (S.58(4)) and the other person must be neither nurse nor doctor (S.58(4)).

It should also be noted that in an emergency, treatment may be given, firstly if it is immediately necessary to save the patient's life, and secondly if it is not irreversible, and it is necessary to alleviate serious suffering by the patient. Thirdly, treatment which is immediately necessary and which represents the minimum interference required to prevent the patient from behaving violently or being a danger to him/herself or others may be given if it is not irreversible or hazardous in nature. 'Irreversible' is defined as treatment entailing unfavourable physical or psychological consequences. 'Hazardous' refers to treatment which entails significant physical hazard.

But is overriding refusal to sanction ECT justifiable? It was noted above that Article 3 does not apply where the treatment is a 'therapeutic necessity'. But what of Article 8, the right to privacy, which can be seen in terms of respect for the autonomy of the individual?

Article 8 is one right which is qualified. Article 8(2) provides that the right may be qualified on the basis of 'the protection of health' where this is 'in accordance with the law and is necessary in a democratic society'. It is possible that any challenge under this Section will be caught by that qualification.

Interestingly, while the prospect of treatment under the Act may be held currently to be lawful, it remains to be seen whether any of the proposals in the new draft Mental Health Bill will be seen to be inconsistent with any of the ECHR principles – in particular, proposals to sanction for the first time compulsory treatment in the community. Davison has argued that 'To avoid breaching Article 8, such orders must also be proportionate to the aim of protecting public health and indeed it is not intended that patients be given medication forcibly, except in a clinical setting' (Davison 2001 at page 199).

As with other areas of practice, dilemmas of consent are often discussed in terms of a conflict of autonomy and best interests. It is sometimes the case, as here, that what professionals think clients/patients need (in terms of treatment, for example), they do not want (Carpenter in Wright & Giddey 1993). In the case of Jack it appears that Articles 2, 3 and 8 would have most relevance. There is also the potential for a conflict of rights should he, for example, continue to refuse treatment which is deemed to be necessary to preserve life.

The right to a therapeutic environment

Case 4b

> *Joanne has been admitted to a mixed sex acute psychiatric ward following a paracetamol overdose. She has a long-standing history of depression, self-harm and alcohol abuse. She was sexually abused by a male relative in childhood. Joanne tells nurses that she does not think she is being helped by the environment. She says the ward is 'shabby' and she does not like sharing facilities with male patients.*

Article 3 (prohibition against torture and inhuman, degrading treatment) has been interpreted as applying to patients in mental hospitals who claim they have been neglected, abused or placed in conditions that are unsanitary or unsafe (Gostin 2000). Individuals or families could, then, claim that when abuse or neglect occurs in hospital or in the community, Article 3 has been violated. It may also be claimed that a violation occurs when the environment is mixed sex or in a poor state of repair. A recent report by MIND concluded that patients/clients in mixed sex psychiatric wards were subject to sexual harassment, abuse and rape (reported in The Guardian 24/02/02). In the case outlined above, Joanne was admitted to a mixed sex ward. Many vulnerable clients, like Joanne, have suffered abuse and a mixed sex environment may not be the most therapeutic environment.

Until recently it was thought that the Article 3 threshold was extremely high and that psychiatric interventions that were a 'therapeutic necessity' could never cross it (Persaud & Hewitt 2001 p.34). It has been pointed out that the Courts have been 'highly deferential to mental health authorities' regarding Article 3 (ibid p.48). In *Herczegfalvy v Austria* (1992) 15 EHRR 437, for example, an individual was admitted to a psychiatric hospital following a hunger strike. He was force fed, attached to a security bed, handcuffed and a belt placed around his ankles due, it was said, to his aggressive behaviour. The Court was concerned about the prolonged use of handcuffs and the security bed but determined that the restraint was medically justified. In another case (*Hilton v United Kingdom* (1978) Application No 5613/72, (1981) 3 EHRR 104, 126) despite claims that a 'mentally disturbed prisoner' was reduced to a state 'like an animal' no violation of Article 3 was found.

A further case brought by MIND in the 1970s in relation to conditions of overcrowding, inadequate sanitary facilities and an atmosphere of violence at Broadmoor hospital failed on the grounds that there was 'no single incident which was so grave as to warrant a finding of inhuman or degrading treatment'. In *Aerts v Belgium* (1999) 5 BHRC 583, A had been detained in the psychiatric wing of a prison because his mental illness was such that he was not criminally responsible and there was no other accommodation. He claimed that the treatment given in the prison hospital amounted to an infringement of Article 3. His claim was however rejected on the facts of the case. The court held that ill-treatment had to have reached a minimum degree of severity and this was an issue to be determined in the light of the facts of the particular case.

However more recently, the case of *Selmouni v France* (1988) 13 EHRR 379 (reported in The Times 24th August) is suggested to have 'lowered the "torture" threshold and might have transformed lesser, hitherto permissible, acts into inhuman and degrading treatment' (Persaud & Hewitt 2001 p.34).

The Ninth Biennial (2001) report from the Mental Health Act Commission highlighted concern about the environment and patients' access to fresh air. The report points out that:

'High priority is given to the need to ensure that patients are placed in the environment best suited to their needs and that security is enhanced by good quality surroundings. Access to activities, fresh air and therapeutic interventions are essential...' (MHAC press release 2001)

In a case such as that of Joanne, above, important questions arise regarding the therapeutic nature of the environment. Is it possible and necessary, for example, to specify minimum standards of environment, treatment and care?

A recent survey of service users by MIND suggests that there is much scope for improvement (Baker/MIND 2000) in care environments for those with mental health problems. The survey found that more than half (56%) of patients surveyed said that wards were 'un-therapeutic' environments and that the ward conditions had a negative effect on their mental health (45%). Thirty per cent of patients found the ward atmosphere 'unsafe and frightening', 'depressing' and bleak (45%). On average, 34% of respondents described the 'overall feeling of the ward' as 'lacking in dignity and respect' (p.10). The report concludes:

'The survey paints a grim picture of life on many psychiatric wards – a depressing environment, unsafe, dirty, with illegal drugs easily available, minimal contact with staff; not enough to do and not enough access to food, drink, bathing facilities, interpreters if needed, telephones and fresh air... Clearly some units are getting it right and there were some warm commendations of wards with good conditions. What people value in these services – for example higher staff:patient ratio, access to the kitchen, service user input at design stage – needs to be built into quality assurance measures for the wider NHS. As well as investment to improve the ward environment, there needs to be a culture change that respects patients and therefore begins by recognising the daily indignities that too many in-patients of acute wards endure.' (Baker/MIND 2000 p.32)

Nurses need to be alert to the therapeutic and non-therapeutic nature of the care environment and ready to take steps to remedy unsatisfactory conditions, where possible. Whilst there is no explicit right to a therapeutic environment in the HRA 1998, Articles 2, 3 and 5 would appear to have particular relevance.

Rights, liberty and security

Case 4c

> *Jason has just taken up a staff nurse position on a unit which caters for the needs of older people with mental health problems. The ward has baffle locks on the doors to prevent the older people leaving the ward and wandering out onto the main road. The majority of the clients are voluntary patients. Jason is concerned about this situation.*

The position of patients such as Jack can be seen in the context of Article 5. Article 5 is a qualified right and states that: 'Everyone has the right to liberty and security of person. No one shall be deprived of his liberty save in the following cases and in accordance with a procedure prescribed by law'. But one of the qualifications to Article 5 provides that:

'(e) the lawful detention of persons for the prevention of infectious diseases, of persons of unsound mind, alcoholics or drug addicts or vagrants.'

The Mental Health Act 1983 provides a legal framework for the lawful detention of patients whose health or safety is in jeopardy or who pose a danger or threat to others. In 1997 the Court of Appeal decided that L, a patient who, due to his severe mental disability, was unable to consent, had been unlawfully detained at Bournewood Hospital. The patient had not been detained under the Mental Health Act 1983 but it was clear that if he had tried to leave, then he would have been. This was deemed unlawful as there was no legal basis for his detention. In 1998 the House of Lords reversed the decision (*R v Bournewood Community and Mental Health NHS Trust, ex parte L* [1998] 3 All ER) (on a three to two majority). Their Lordships differed over the issue as to whether L was actually detained. Lord Steyn and Lord Nolan took the approach that while L was detained, this detention was sanctioned under the common law.

It may thus be the case that a person without capacity may be admitted under common law and de facto detained even though the provisions of the Mental Health Act 1983 have not been complied with.

Case 4c highlights a possible conflict between the client/patient's right to liberty and the staff duty of care. It might also be argued that the right to liberty and the right to security are at odds in a case such as this. It might be claimed that baffle locks to prevent clients from leaving the unit and walking onto, for example, a busy road, violated the right to freedom but supported the right to security. There are further issues of voluntariness in psychiatric wards, as in the Bournewood case. Are clients 'voluntary', for example, if staff threaten them with MHA detention should they attempt to leave? In the case outlined here, it is important that those who are sufficiently competent are not detained unlawfully. Baffle locks are a form of restraint and should only be used when there is no satisfactory alternative. If baffle locks are used as a means to, for example, cut staffing levels then the therapeutic nature of the environment is in question.

As far as detention through the use of locked doors in such a situation is concerned, the Code of Practice provides:

> 'The safety of informal patients who would be at risk of harm if they wandered out of a ward or mental nursing at home at will, should be ensured by adequate staffing and good supervision. Combination locks and double handed doors should be used only in units where there is a regular and significant risk of patients wandering off accidentally and being at risk of harm. There should be clear policies on the use of locks and other devices and a mechanism for reviewing decisions. Every patient should have an individual care plan which states explicitly when he or she will be prevented from leaving the ward. Patients who are not deliberately trying to leave the ward, but who may wander out accidentally, may legitimately be deterred from leaving the ward by those devices. In the case of a patient who persistently and/or purposely attempts to leave a ward or mental nursing home, whether or not they understand the risk involved, considerations must be given to assessing whether they would more appropriately be formally detained...' (Code of Practice para 19.27)

The Bournewood case has now been referred to the European Court of Human Rights. Article 5 clearly highlights the importance of 'a procedure prescribed by law' so it is unclear if the Bournewood decision will stand (Fennell 1998). Indeed it has been suggested that the ECHR would militate in favour of a different result on the same facts in such a situation, and that the approach in *Ashingdane v UK* ((1985) 7 EHRR 528) requires consideration of

> 'the concrete situation of the individual concerned and account must be taken of a whole range of criteria such as the type, duration, effect and manner of implementation of the measure in question.'

Ashingdane was held in an open ward but still detained. In other cases much seems to turn on their particular facts (*W v Sweden* Application No 127778/87 and *L v Sweden* Application No 10801/84).

Should detention on this basis be deemed incompatible with the Human Rights Act 1998? It has been estimated that some 22,000 patients in a similar position in hospital would require a formal assessment (ibid) under the Mental Health Act 1983. It might be argued, as Lord Steyn did, that there would be advantages in terms of additional safeguards from these patients being sectioned under the Mental Health Act 1983.

The Mental Health Act Draft Bill now provides that persons with long-term incapacity who are not sectioned under the legislation will have enhanced rights. These include the appointment of a 'nominated person' to act on their behalf, treatment on the basis of an agreed care plan, access to specialist advocacy and, most importantly in the light of the ECHR, the ability to challenge their admission and treatment before the Mental Health Tribunal (Department of Health 2002).

Right to a fair trial

Case 4d

> *Amos is a 24-year-old man who describes himself as Afro-Caribbean. He has been admitted to an acute ward and is detained under Section 2 of the Mental Health Act. Staff took the view that his mental health state was deteriorating as he admitted to hearing voices. Amos argues that his life may not be as orderly as many other people's but that he is managing fine. He asks his named nurse how he might challenge his detention and asks if she will speak for him. He says that he fears that his British psychiatrist does not understand him.*

Amos is detained under Section 2 of the Act. The Mental Health Act enables a trust or health authority to discharge any patient who has been admitted for assessment or treatment at any time (Section 23). The decision to discharge is to be taken by a committee of three persons (Sections 24(4) and 24(5)). A patient also has the right to apply for discharge to a Mental Health Review Tribunal (Section 66). An automatic reference will be made to a tribunal where the patient has not exercised the right to apply during the first six months of detention, and an automatic referral must be made if the patient has not been before the tribunal for three years. A Mental Health Review Tribunal (of which there are eight nationally) is composed of three members: one legal, one medical and one lay. It is required to discharge patients where they are no longer suffering from mental disorder/illness or where further detention is not required for the purposes of the patient's health or safety or to protect other persons. The tribunal also has a discretion to discharge, even where the criteria have not been satisfied.

Several provisions of the ECHR are relevant here. Article 5(4) provides that:

'Everyone who is deprived of his liberty by arrest or detention shall be entitled to take proceedings by which the lawfulness of his detention shall be decided speedily by a court and his release ordered if his detention is not lawful.'

Article 6 (right to a fair trial) states that:

'In the determination of his civil rights and obligations or of any criminal charge against him, everyone is entitled to a fair and public hearing within a reasonable time by an independent and impartial tribunal established by law.'

The operation of Mental Health Review Tribunals has been the subject of challenge in a number of recent human rights cases. We noted in Chapter 1 the amendment made to the burden of proof in relation to individuals making applications for discharge in such cases which led to the first declaration of incompatibility (*R v MHRT North and East London Region and another ex parte H* [2001] EWCA Civ 415). One issue regarding tribunals is the extent to which they can be seen as adequately independent bodies. The role of the medical member of the tribunal has been criticised. It has been suggested that he is influential and that his role is not subject to cross-examination (Davison 2001 at page 182). However, in *R (on the application of H) v MHR Tribunal to North and East London Region* [2000] WL 1720256 the argument that the tribunal contravened Article 5(4), as medical members were both expert witnesses and decision makers, was rejected. Indeed comparisons were drawn with the effective operation of inquisitorial systems in other European countries. Nonetheless Crane J went on to emphasise that there did need to be 'equality of arms' and that:

> 'if the medical member is taking into account or is drawing to the attention of other members either evidence or his views as an expert, then the claimant and his advisers should be alerted to such evidence and such views in sufficient detail and sufficiently early in the proceedings to enable them to deal with them.'

While this case was later overturned on appeal this issue was not explicitly dealth with.

Applications must also be dealt with 'speedily', and while this is not defined in *R (on the application of C) v MHRT London South and South West Region* (2001) a policy which had held that applications would be heard within 8 weeks was held to be unlawful under the Human Rights Act. Such specific time limits should not be enforced where a more rapid review date was practicable. In a recent High Court ruling, the government was found to have breached the human rights of seven people who were detained under the Mental Health Act 1983 (*R The Queen on the Applications of KB, MK, JR, GM, LB, PD and TB v The Mental Health Review Tribunal, The Secretary of State for Health* [2002] EWHC 639, 2002 K52 NLJ 672). Here the seven successfully claimed that they did not receive speedy reviews by the Mental Health Review Tribunals. In each case the hearing arranged by the tribunal was adjourned repeatedly and the delays ranged from 9 weeks 5 days to over 22 weeks.

In mental health the connection between, and crucial importance of, Articles 5 and 6 is clear. Mental health legislation can legitimately deprive individuals of their liberty. An independent and efficient mechanism is essential to ensure that those who are detained have a means to challenge their detention. The recent case referred to above has highlighted shortcomings in the Mental Health Review Tribunal system and the implications for patients and staff have been highlighted.

Article 14 is concerned with the prohibition of discrimination in relation to the 'enjoyment of the rights and freedoms' outlined in the HRA 1998. In 2000, the Mental Health Act Commission reported evidence of 'race bias in mental health wards' (Brindle 2000). The Commission found that only a small number of those who spoke little or no English were provided with an interpreter. Lack of appropriate interpreting services could, for example, jeopardise a patient/client's right to a fair hearing as required by Article 6 discussed above.

There have also been reports of differences in detention rates and in treatment options offered to those in non-white groups. Non-white groups, particularly Afro-Caribbeans, are more likely to be detained and to be given treatments such as drugs and electro-convulsive therapy rather than psychotherapy (ibid). Article 3 might also be relevant here in relation to Article 14.

Under the proposed reforms of the Mental Health Act, it is intended that the tribunal will have a far larger role in sanctioning decision making. This will lead to an increased workload, and concerns have been expressed as to whether there are sufficient clinical personnel available to operate these bodies. The Government is presently consulting as to whether a single person tribunal may be capable of operating in some situations (Draft Bill: Consultation Document 2002). It will of course be of even greater importance, given the enhanced role of the tribunal, to ensure that it operates effectively within the scope of the ECHR.

Conclusion

Human rights and mental health are inextricably linked and the case law of the ECHR graphically illustrates just some of the interfaces.

It seems likely that many more such cases will come through the courts in the future. An awareness of some of the central rights issues in mental health practice better prepares nurses to work with this particularly vulnerable client group.

A number of rights were identified which appear to have most relevance. Article 2 highlights the importance of having systematic risk assessment procedures in place and ensuring that sufficient provision has been made to prevent suicide attempts. Article 3 draws attention to many of the possible issues in practice which may be considered degrading or inhuman. Issues such as mixed sex wards, which the government is already committed to phasing out (see http://www/doh.gov.uk/mhmixedaccom.htm), and physical treatments will need to be continually evaluated in relation to Article 3. The recent MIND report 'Environmentally Friendly?' (Baker/MIND 2000) suggests that there is some way to go in the achievement of a therapeutic and respectful environment for all.

An appreciation of Articles 5 and 6 is particularly crucial as mental health practice allows for the deprivation of an individual's freedom and requires that they have a fair and speedy hearing should they wish their detention to be reconsidered. Article 8 is likely to have many consequences in practice. In the light of the continuing stigma attached to mental illness, individuals will be keen to ensure that their right to privacy is maintained. Awareness of the limitations on this right is important. Other privacy considerations include the use of CCTV and search policies. As with other areas of practice, there is the potential for conflict within and amongst the rights specified in the HRA 1998. It may be, for example, that there is tension between the individual's right to liberty and to security – allowing the individual freedom may jeopardise his and others' security should he suffer from a serious mental health problem.

Respecting the individual's right to privacy by not implementing a search policy may compromise his right to life if, for example, s/he is concealing the means (drugs, sharp objects) to take her/his own life. Article 10 (freedom of expression) has been highlighted as relevant to mental health practice but is not discussed here. Persaud & Hewitt (2001) suggest the possible implications of Article 10 in relation to, for example, the distribution of material which is not considered appropriate to be viewed by an individual patient or patient group. Article 14 cannot be viewed in isolation as it refers to non-discrimination in relation to the exercise of other rights in the HRA 1998. It is important to ensure that within practice respect for the rights discussed is not variable amongst those of different ethnic backgrounds, age or gender.

As with other areas of practice, there is much here which remains tentative. It continues to be important for nurses in this particularly challenging area to reflect on the meaning of the Articles discussed here and to consider how best to promote such rights in practice.

As some of the examples and decided cases illustrate, the existing law may be regarded as problematic when considering the application of the Mental Health Act. In terms of the proposed new Mental Health Act, there may be additional issues which challenge legislators and practitioners committed to rights in practice.

References

Baker S, MIND 2000 Environmentally friendly? Patients' views of conditions on psychiatric wards. MIND, London

Bartlett P, Sandland R 2000 Mental health policy law and practice. Blackstones, London

Batty D 2001 ECT practitioners and users welcome review. The Guardian 29/08/02

Brindle D 2000 Spot check finds race bias in mental wards. The Guardian 06/03/02

British Medical Association 1992 Medicine betrayed. Zed Books, London

British Medical Association 2001 The medical profession & human rights – Handbook for a changing agenda. Zed Books in association with the BMA, London

Carpenter D 1993 In the best interests of the client? Legal and ethical principles. In: Wright H, Giddey H (eds) Mental health nursing: From first principles to professional practice. Chapman & Hall, London

Coombes L 1998 Mental health. In: Chadwick R (ed) Encyclopaedia of applied ethics, volume 3. Academic Press, San Diego

Davison L 2001 The impact of the Human Rights Act 1998 on mental health law, parts I and II. In: Garwood-Gowers A, Tingle J, Lewis T (eds) Healthcare law: The impact of the Human Rights Act 1998. Cavendish, London

Department of Health 1999 National service framework for mental health. HMSO, London

Department of Health Reform of the Mental Health Act 1983: proposals for consultations. Cm 4480

Department of Health and Welsh Office 1999 Code of practice – Mental Health Act 1983. HMSO, London

Department of Health 2000 Safety, privacy and dignity in mental health units – Guidance on mixed sex accommodation for mental health services. http://www.doh.gov.uk/mhmixedsexaccom.htm

Department of Health 2002 Mental health draft bill http://www.doh.gov.uk/mentalhealth/draftbill2002

Fennell P 1998 Doctor knows best? Therapeutic detention under common law, the Mental Health Act and the European Convention. Medical Law Review 6: 32

Fennell P 2002 Detention of untreatable psychopaths and Article 5 of the ECHR. Medical Law Review: 92

Fulford K W M 1998 Mental illness, concept of health. In: Chadwick R (ed) Encyclopaedia of applied ethics, volume 3. Academic Press, San Diego

General Assembly of the United Nations 1991 The protection of persons with mental illness and the improvement of mental health care http://www.un.org/documents/ga/res/46/a46r119.htm

Glover-Thomas N 2002 Reconstructing mental health law and policy law in context. Butterworths, London

Goffman E 1961 Asylums. Doubleday & Co, Anchor Books, New York

Gostin L O 2000 Human rights of persons with mental disabilities - the EHCR. International Journal of Law & Psychiatry 23 (2): 125

The Guardian (Society section) 2002 Psychiatric patients abused on mixed-sex wards. The Guardian 24/04/02

Halpern A L, Freedman A M 2000 Eternal vigilance is the price of human rights. Mental Health Reform 5:1

Laing J Care or custody: mentally disordered offenders in the criminal justice system. Oxford University Press, Oxford

Lord Chancellor's Department 1999 Making Decisions. LCD, London

Mann J M, Gostin L, Gruskin S et al 1999 Health and human rights. In: Mann J M, Gruskin S, Grodin M A et al (eds) Health and human rights – A reader. Routledge, New York and London

Mental Health Act Commission 2001 Ninth Biennial Report. Mental Health Act Commission, Nottingham

NHS 1999 National service framework for mental health. Stationery Office, London

NMC 2002 Code of professional conduct. Nursing & Midwifery Council, London

Persaud A, Hewitt D 2001 European Convention on Human Rights: Effects on psychiatric care. Nursing Standard 1 (44): 33-37

Richardson G 1999 Report of the Expert Committee review of the Mental health Act 1983. Department of Health, London

UKCC 1998 Guidelines for mental health and learning disabilities nursing – A guide to working with vulnerable clients. United Kingdom Central for Nursing, Midwifery and Health Visiting, London

UKCC 2000 The nursing, midwifery and health visiting contribution to the continuing care of people with mental health problems – A review and UKCC action plan. United Kingdom Central Council for Nursing, Midwifery and Health Visiting, London

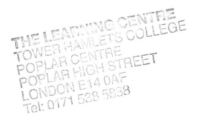

Chapter 5

The right to privacy and health information

Introduction

Nurses, midwives and health visitors have privileged access to personal information and to the persons/bodies of patients. How they manage such information and approach personal care activities has the potential to enhance or inhibit the development of a trusting patient-professional relationship.

Technological and research developments in health care such as genetics and information technology urge an ongoing consideration of safeguards to promote privacy in practice. Privacy is connected with, and yet distinguishable from, values such as confidentiality, autonomy and dignity. Patient confidentiality has historically long been recognised as part of clinical practice. The Hippocratic Oath, for example, stated:

'Whatever, in connection with my professional practice, or not in connection with it, I see or hear, in the life of men, which ought not to be spoken of abroad, I will not divulge, as reckoning that all such should be kept secret.'

A right to privacy has been traced back to 1890 and the writings of the US jurists Warren and Brandeis (Warren & Brandeis 1890) when it was equated with the 'right to be left alone' (Woogara 2001 p.237). The right to privacy has now been bolstered by Article 8 of the ECHR. Article 8 of the HRA 1998 sets out the right to privacy of home and family life.

Arguably the effect of Article 8 is to go beyond simply acting as a 'bolster'; it may be seen as a means of redefining the boundaries of health information privacy. It has been used to confirm individual control rights over information whether in the form of restraining access or enabling an individual to obtain access to their information (*Gaskin v UK* (1989) 12 EHRR 36). Concerns regarding the need to safeguard privacy can be seen behind the EU Data Protection Directive and the subsequent passage of the UK Data Protection Act 1998 which provides legislative safeguards regarding the control of information held on computer and also on manual files.

The Data Protection Act 1998 applies to health information that identifies a living individual including that which is recorded in electronic and manual health records (S.1(1)). Health records include records which are part of an organised filing system (S.68(2)) and also any other kind of record that consists of information relating to the physical or mental health condition of an individual or made by or on behalf of a health professional in connection with the care of that individual (S.68(2)). Health professionals include doctors, nurses, health visitors, clinical psychologists, child psychotherapists, dentists, opticians and pharmacists (S.69). Schedule 1 of the Act sets out eight data protection principles that must be observed by persons who process personal data. The first principle of Schedule 1 requires data be processed in a fair and lawful manner. The processing must comply with one of the conditions set forth in Schedule 2. Health information is defined as 'sensitive personal data' (S.2) and must also meet one of the conditions in Schedule 3 of the Act. Schedule 2 sets out the types of situations when personal data may be processed or disclosed to other persons. Information may be divulged with the consent of the data subject, in compliance with a legal obligation to which the data controller is subject (e.g. statutory reporting requirements), or when disclosure is in the 'vital interests' of the data subject. Schedule 2 also allows data processing for the legitimate purposes of the data controller or third parties provided it does not 'prejudice' the rights, freedoms or legitimate interests of the data subject.

In addition to meeting one of the conditions of Schedule 2, processing of health information must also meet at least one of the conditions set out in Schedule 3. Paragraph 8 of this schedule sanctions disclosure when necessary for 'medical purposes', provided it is carried out by a health professional who owes a duty of confidentiality or other person who owes a similar duty. 'Medical purposes' include preventative medicine, medical research, the provision of care and of treatment and management of health care services. Information may also be disclosed under Paragraph 3 of Schedule 3, where disclosure is made to protect the 'vital interests' of a subject who is unable to consent, or whose consent cannot reasonably be obtained. The schedule also provides that information may be disclosed where the consent has been unreasonably withheld and disclosure is necessary to protect the vital interests of another person.

In addition the remaining data protection principles provide that, under principle 2, personal data shall be obtained only for one or more specified and lawful purposes, and shall not be further processed in any manner incompatible with that purpose or those purposes. Principle 3 provides that personal data shall be adequate, relevant, and not excessive in relation to the purpose or purposes for which they are processed. Principle 4 states that personal data shall be accurate and, where necessary, kept up to date. Principle 5 provides that personal data processed for any purpose or purposes shall not be kept for longer than is necessary for that purpose or those purposes. Principle 6 notes that personal data shall be processed in accordance with the rights of data subjects under this Act. Principle 7 states that appropriate technical and organisational measures shall be taken against unauthorised or unlawful processing of personal data and against accidental loss or destruction of, or damage to, personal data. Finally principle 8 provides that personal data shall not be transferred to a country or territory outside the European Economic Area unless that country or territory ensures an adequate level of protection for the rights and freedoms of data subjects in relation to the processing of personal data.

The data protection principles are subject to enforcement by the Information Commissioner. In addition, a data subject may ask that incorrect information be rectified (S.14), claim compensation for damages and distress (S.13) and prevent processing of data which is likely to occasion distress or damages (S.10).

The data subject may apply for access to information about them under Section 7 of the 1998 Act. Such information must be supplied 'promptly' and within 40 days. The individual may be required to pay a fee, subject to a statutory maximum. Access to health care records may be withheld if the information may cause serious harm to the physical or mental health or condition of the data subject or any other person (Data Protection (Subject Access Modification) (Health) Order 2000 SI 2000/413, art. 5). Information can be withheld where this would otherwise lead to disclosure of information relating to an identifiable third party. There is an exception where the third party has given his or her consent, or when it is reasonable under the circumstances to disclose without consent (S.7(4)).

Particularly importantly, this legislation operates alongside the existing law concerning confidentiality and privacy and does not supersede it – it simply complements it.

Similarly such concerns led to the establishment of the Caldicott Committee whose report led to the establishment of Caldicott guardians in the NHS (Caldicott 1997). These are responsible for the documentation of the use of person-identifiable information (NHSE 1999).

The Nursing and Midwifery Council Code of Professional Conduct (NMC 2002) does not refer to privacy explicitly but does discuss confidentiality. Section 5 states that:

'As a registered nurse, midwife or health visitor, you must protect confidential information'

and

'You must treat information about patients and clients as confidential and use it only for the purposes for which it was given. As it is impractical to obtain consent every time you need to share information with others, you should ensure that patients and clients understand that some information may be made available to other members of the team involved in the delivery of care. You must guard against breaches of confidentiality by protecting from improper disclosure at all times.'

The NMC points to situations where information can be shared with others: with the patient's consent; or without the patient's consent in two circumstances – in the public interest and where required by law or court order. Adherence to child protection policies is highlighted and confidentiality must be in accord with these.

The significance of privacy in health care has been acknowledged in the NHS Plan 2000 in relation to older people:

'Wherever older people are cared for, we will expect that both they and their carers will be treated in a way which respects their dignity, privacy and autonomy. This is not an addition to care provision, it is an integral part of good care.' (Department of Health 2000 p.129)

It is, of course, not the case that privacy relates only to one specific client group although privacy violations have been more apparent here (see, for example, National Service Framework for Older People (2002) Standard 2; HAS 2000 (1998) 'Not Because They Are Old'; and Counsel and Care (1991) 'Not Such Private Places'). Media reports relating to other areas of health care highlight the devastating impact of professional breaches of patient privacy (see, for example, Dutter in The Telegraph 25/04/97 'GP's drunken betrayal left our lives in tatters').

In this chapter we focus upon the boundaries of disclosure regarding control and disclosure of information in general but not the question of patient access to records. Readers are referred to other commentators (Kennedy & Grubb 2000; Stone 2002; Montgomery 2002). First, we will discuss some definitional issues, arguments to support privacy, and the background to the right to privacy.

The word 'privacy' is said to have its roots in the Latin *privatus* which means literally 'belongs to oneself' (Glen & Jownally 1995). A number of approaches have been taken to 'privacy'. Laurie refers to it as being a 'separateness from others' (Laurie 2002 p.6). Allen (in Beauchamp & Childress 2001 p.294-5) distinguishes four forms of privacy:

- informational privacy, which relates to information
- physical privacy, which relates to individuals and their personal spaces
- decisional privacy, which concerns the individual's choices, and

- proprietary privacy, which concerns 'property interests in the human person'.

Beauchamp and Childress (2001 p.295) add a fifth form of privacy: relational or associational privacy, which acknowledges family and other intimate relationships and the fact that individuals make decisions within these relationships. On this account, a loss of privacy occurs 'if others use any of several forms of access, including intervening in zones of secrecy, anonymity, seclusion or solitude' (ibid p.295). While the right to privacy recognised under Article 8 extends potentially to the range of 'privacy rights' highlighted above, in this chapter we are mostly concerned with the category known as 'informational privacy'.

The need for information privacy or confidentiality within health care is crucial. As Woogara (2001 p.240) puts it:

'Informational privacy allows patients the right to control information about them, even after divulging it to carers. This component acknowledges the critical value of patients being able to step forward and participate in their own care in the full knowledge that any information about themselves and their identity released to health professionals will be protected.'

Three main types of argument are presented for safeguarding the confidentiality of patient information (Ngwena & Chadwick 1994) – a duty-based argument; an autonomy-based argument; and the argument from utility. Duty-based or deontological arguments are evident in professional codes. The view is that preserving confidentiality is something we have a duty to do, based on an intuition that this is a good thing in itself and also based on 'an implied promise in the professional-client relationship' (ibid p.139). Autonomy has been identified as a key principle in health care ethics (see, for example, Chapter 3 in Beauchamp & Childress 2001; Gillon 1994; Dworkin 1988). Autonomy literally means 'self-rule' or self-determination. It concerns our ability and, some would say, our right to have control over our lives. Part of this control relates to the management of personal information. As Ngwena and Chadwick put it:

'Those who believe there is an obligation to promote the autonomy of patients and clients, in the sense of self-determination, have a reason to uphold the view that confiders of personal information to health professionals should be free to decide whether such information should be divulged further. On a wider interpretation... it may be argued that to have control over information about oneself is a necessary condition of having a life that one can call one's own.' (ibid p.139)

The third argument is based on utility. According to a utilitarian argument, actions are right to the extent they promote good consequences and wrong to the extent they contribute to bad consequences. Where patients are aware that confidentiality is maintained, it is more likely that they will share information relevant to their health status. If confidentiality is not maintained then they may hold back from seeking care or be insufficiently candid regarding the information which they do ultimately provide through fear of stigma or of discrimination. As Gillon (1995 p.108) states:

'people's better health, welfare, the general good and overall happiness are more likely to be attained if doctors (and we would add, nurses) are fully informed by their patients, and this is more likely if doctors undertake not to disclose patients' secrets.'

(See also Gillon 1994 'Medical Ethics: Four Principles Plus Attention to Scope' – here he makes virtually the same point.)

There is no general overarching protection in English law for the privacy of patient information through a single statute. Instead, confidentiality is maintained through the application of what is known as the equitable remedy of breach of confidence and through certain specific statutory provisions, for example, in relation to venereal disease, infertility treatment (through the Human Fertilisation and Embryology Act 1990). In law the need for confidentiality has been seen as self-evident (*Ashworth v MGN* [2001] 1 All ER 991). Confidentiality has however never been recognised in absolute terms and there are a series of statutory exceptions, for example in relation to notifiable diseases (under the Public Health Act), or regarding the treatment of drug addicts (Misuse of Drugs (Notification of Supply to Addicts) Regulations 1973 SI 1973 No 799) or where information is required in relation to judicial proceedings (*AG v Mulholland* [1962] 2 QB 477).

There have been a small number of cases which indicate how the European Court of Human Rights itself regards claims regarding Article 8 in a health care context. In *MS v Sweden* (1997) 45 BMLR 133 the applicant failed to convince the ECHR that her right to private life had been infringed. It was held that the State Insurance Office (SIO) had had a legitimate interest in obtaining her medical records from her clinic, without her prior consent, in response to her claim for a disability pension. The Court recognised, in particular, the need to protect the public purse from abuse through fraud. This could only be done with access to relevant information and the applicant was in no position to restrict the availability of that information in the circumstances. The Court noted that there were adequate safeguards under legislation which prevented that information from being misused by the SIO. From this case, it can therefore be assumed that Article 8 will not be breached

- where a state body has a legitimate interest in obtaining medical information
- where that information is being obtained as a corollary to an applicant initiated-claim for a benefit, and
- where there are adequate safeguards for confidentiality.

In *Z v Finland* (1997) 25 EHRR 371 (Ect HR) the issue concerned disclosure of a person's HIV positive status. Z's husband was tried for a number of sexual offences, and for attempted manslaughter. One issue was whether he knew that he was HIV positive at the time of the offences.

Disclosure of Z's medical records was sought as Z invoked her right not to give evidence. While the court made an order guaranteeing the confidentiality of the proceedings, this was only guaranteed for 10 years. The European Court of Human Rights noted the need to safeguard the privacy of health information, particularly in relation to something such as HIV which so crucially concerned confidential information. However, there were also public policy considerations such as that of safeguarding the public against crime and disorder. They held that orders requiring her medical advisors to give evidence and in relation to the seizure of the medical records were justifiable and outweighed her Article 8 claim. However, interestingly, the Court was of the view that the order making the medical records available to the public after ten years did not sufficiently protect her right to private and family life and here the Court found a violation of Article 8.

This case was followed by the English courts in *A Health Authority v X* [2001] 2 FLR 673 where the court allowed disclosure of clinical records to a health authority investigating GPs to determine whether they had complied with their terms of service. While this disclosure was held to be legitimate, the scope of the disclosure was limited for those purposes which were stated.

Prior to the Human Rights Act in 1998, in a series of cases the English courts had stated that the right to privacy was not part of English law (*Kaye v Robertson* [1991] FSR 62; *Malone v MPC* [1979] 2 All ER 620). Since the Act came into force in 2000 the courts have had the tools to fashion such a right. In *Douglas v Hello* ([2001] 2 WLR 992) Sedley LJ stated that 'we have now reached a point at which it can be said with confidence that the law recognises and will appropriately protect a right of personal privacy.' He commented that this right was rooted in the equitable remedy of breach of confidence.

Also in *Venables v Newsgroup Newspapers* [2001] 2 WLR 1038, which concerned publication of information which could lead to the identification of the applicants who had been convicted of the murder of the infant James Bulger, Dame Butler Sloss held that in granting relief this could again be seen as 'an extension of the law of breach of confidence'. Here the injunction was granted not only on the basis of Article 8 – and the court indicated that it was uncertain as to whether an injunction would have been granted on the basis of Article 8 itself – but also on the basis of Articles 2 and 3.

It appears that currently, in the context of health care the courts will consider the question of privacy from the backdrop of health care confidentiality (*R v Department of Health ex parte Source Informatics Ltd* [2000] 1 All ER 786 CA) (see below).

Patients' rights to privacy and confidentiality

Case 5a

> *Susan has been admitted to hospital for investigations as she had symptoms*
> *of extreme weight loss and fatigue. On admission Susan tells her named*
> *nurse that when the results become available she does not want her husband*
> *to be given this information.*

The health care professionals caring for Susan are obliged to maintain confidentiality – firstly, because this is required under their professional ethical codes and breach of confidence may lead to disciplinary action. Secondly, confidentiality is likely to be a stipulation under their contract of employment. Finally, confidentiality is also safeguarded through the application of the equitable remedy of breach of confidence.

The equitable remedy of breach of confidence provides that where information is entrusted subject to an obligation of confidence – whether express or implied – then unauthorised disclosure of such information constitutes a breach of confidence. The grounds on which an action for breach of confidence may be brought are set out in *AG v Guardian Newspapers* [1988] 3 All ER 545 at 658 by Lord Goff:

> '... a duty of confidence arises where confidential information comes to the knowledge of a person (the confidant) in circumstances where he has notice or is held to have agreed that the information is confidential with the effect that it would be just in all the circumstances where he should be precluded from disclosing the information to others.'

Such an obligation of confidentiality will arise in the context of a health care practitioner-patient relationship such as doctor-patient or nurse-patient. So for example in *X v Y* in 1988 a national newspaper wanted to publish details regarding two GPs who were HIV positive. Rose J held that:

> 'In the long run preservation of confidentiality is the only way of securing public health: otherwise doctors would be discredited as a source of education, for future patients will not come forward if doctors are going to squeal on them. Consequently confidentiality is vital to secure public as well as private health, for unless those infected come forward they cannot be counselled and self-treatment does not provide the best care: opportunistic infections such as shortness of breath and signs of disease in the nervous system (including dementia from HIV encephalopathy) are better detected and responded to by observation, investigation and management in hospital.'

In law, however, the obligation of confidentiality is not absolute. The House of Lords in *AG v Guardian Newspapers* confirmed that the court needed to undertake a balancing test between the public interest in the maintenance of confidentiality and the public interest in disclosure. In constructing what amounts to public interest in disclosure the courts have taken note of professional practice guidelines such as those issued by the General Medical Council (*X v Y* [1988] 2 All ER 648; *W v Egdell* [1989] 1 All ER 1089; *Woolgar v Chief Constable of Sussex* [1999] 3 All ER 604 etc.). Most recently they have also construed exceptions to confidentiality in terms of Article 8.

In *R v Department of Health ex parte Source Informatics* [2000] 1 All ER 786 the court took a different approach. This case concerned disclosure of anonymised data concerning GPs' prescribing habits to a firm who wanted the information to sell to pharmaceutical companies. Here the Court of Appeal held that there was no breach of confidence on the basis that 'The concern of the law here is to protect the confider's personal privacy. That and that alone is the right at issue in the confider's personal privacy.' In this particular situation the view was taken that there was no threat to privacy, because the information was anonymised. The court also looked at the effect that the obligation of confidentiality had on the 'conscience' of the pharmacist. In this case their view was that a reasonable pharmacist's conscience 'would not be troubled by the proposed use made of patients' prescriptions'. This case has been subject to criticism. Laurie, for example, argues that to suggest that there is no breach of confidence where there is no unfairness to the confider implies that this may be so even where the use is unauthorised (Laurie 2002 at page 225). He also criticises this case because it removes the 'public interest' criteria. He argues that 'this is particularly disturbing because it also led the court to ignore the wider and longer term impact of its decision on the public interest in maintaining confidences generally' (page 225). The case has been subject to criticism on other grounds. Beyleveld and Histed have commented that:

> 'a patient may object to Source Informatics scheme because he or she has deep personal ethical concerns about contributing to the profit making of large pharmaceutical manufacturers based on knowledge of those manufacturers' lack of ethical concerns in other, less advanced countries.' (Beyleveld & Histed 2000)

This case, as Laurie notes, is an exception and indeed, as he notes, it does not affect the position once a duty has been accepted to exist.

In the example before us the patient has a right to ensure that there is no unauthorised disclosure of personal information, and that right is undoubtedly bolstered by the right to privacy. In Susan's case there seems to be good reason to assume that her right to privacy should be safeguarded. The exceptions regarding confidentiality as outlined in the NMC Code 2002 do not seem to apply – she has not given consent for the disclosure of information to her family; there is no public interest as far as we know, and no court order.

Overiding privacy/confidentiality in the public interest

Case 5b

> *James is an in-patient on a secure psychiatric unit and has submitted an appeal to the Mental Health Review Tribunal to review his detention under Section 3 of the Mental Health Act 1983. His named nurse, Liz, is required to submit a report. In one of their regular care plan meetings, James asks Liz not to disclose the information he has shared with her as this is 'confidential'. Some weeks before, James had disclosed that he had 'murderous' thoughts relating to his parents.*

The English courts, as noted above, have been prepared to balance out the public interest in maintaining confidentiality versus the public interest in maintaining that confidentiality. In 1989, Dr Egdell (*W v Edgell* [1989] 1 All ER 1089) was commissioned to prepare a report for solicitors concerning a patient, W, who was held in hospital under a restriction order. W's case was due to come before a Mental Health Review Tribunal. The report commissioned by Dr Egdell was not favourable and in the light of the report the solicitors decided to withdraw the case from the tribunal. Dr Egdell asked the solicitors to forward a copy of the report to the hospital but they refused. Subsequently, W's case came for automatic review before a Mental Health Review Tribunal. A copy of the report was circulated to the Home Office and the Hospital. W's solicitors brought an action for breach of confidence. However in the Court of Appeal it was held that Dr Egdell was justified in his disclosure as it was in the public interest. Bingham LJ stated that:

> 'Where a man has committed multiple killings under the disability of serious mental illness, decisions which may lead directly or indirectly to his release from hospital should not be made unless a responsible authority is properly able to make an informed judgment that the risk of repetition is so small as to be acceptable. A consultant psychiatrist who becomes aware, even in the course of a confidential relationship, of information which leads him, in the exercise of what the court considers a sound professional judgment, to fear that such decisions may be made on the basis of inadequate information and with a real risk of consequent danger to the public is entitled to take such steps as are reasonable in all the circumstances to communicate the grounds of his concern to the responsible authorities.'

At first instance in this case the judge even suggested that a doctor in such a situation may be under a 'duty' to disclose such information.

In *R v Crozier* [1990] 8 BMLR 128 Crozier had been detained in hospital under a restriction order after trial for attempted murder. Dr M was instructed to make a report for the defence. Although he did so, the report itself did not arrive in time for the hearing. Dr M arrived just as the judge was passing sentence. He informed the barrister for the Crown that C was suffering from a mental illness of a psychopathic nature and that he should be detained in a maximum secure unit. The Crown appealed and obtained variation of sentence. The defence in turn then appealed on the basis that the disclosure made by Dr M was in breach of confidence. Watkins LJ held that it was clearly in the public interest for this information to be disclosed and that this was particularly important in view of the fact that Dr M knew that a Dr W who had initially seen C and had been of the view that he was not suffering from a mental disorder had changed his mind. It should be noted that the courts have distinguished what amounts to the 'public interest' from what is interesting to the public to know (*Lion Laboratories v Evans* [1984] 2 All ER 417).

This public interest justification in disclosure is echoed in the rulings of the European Court of Human Rights. In *TV v Finland* (Case No 21780/93 76A DR 140) it was held by the Commission that disclosure of the HIV positive status of a prisoner to prison staff was justifiable as this was necessary for protection of health. In this particular instance however the prison staff were subject to obligations of confidentiality. They were also persons involved directly with the prisoner.

In such cases the health care professional can be involved in what are highly problematic issues of risk assessment. Here the interface between maintaining the privacy of the individual is balanced against considerations of prevention of crime and disorder. The patient may pose a risk to others. But at what point does this risk cede to the rights of others? As Mason notes:

'The accurate assessment of the risk of dangerous behaviour seems to be a near impossibility and is, at best, a highly subjective exercise.' (Mason 2000, p.69)

There is already a considerable amount of literature on the issue of whether the health care professional will be held liable if they actually fail to break confidentiality in a particular situation. The leading case is a US case, that of *Tarasoff v Regents of the University of California* (551 p.2d 334 (Cal.1976)) in which a patient confided in his therapist that he intended to kill the woman, Miss Tarasoff, who had rejected his advances. His therapist reported him to the University Campus police; they detained him but then decided to release him. Miss Tarasoff came back from vacation and the patient killed her. The court said that there was in a situation, as here, a special relationship between therapist and patient such that this was sufficient to create a duty to exercise reasonable care. The English courts have however never recognised a *Tarasoff* duty and indeed they are unwilling to extend liability regarding the actions of third parties (*Osman v Ferguson* [1993] 4 All ER 344 and *Palmer v Tees HA* [1999] Lloyds Rep Med 351).

There are a number of challenges which face nurses in cases such as that of James. On the one hand the nurse has her obligation to act as the patient's advocate and to respect his privacy under Article 8. On the other hand Article 8 is a right which is qualified by public interest considerations. There is also the extent to which Article 2 (the right to life of others) may be regarded as being applicable in this situation.

Where that balance lies will vary from case to case. In some cases the patient may be simply voicing feelings which they have absolutely no intention whatsoever of actualising as conduct. If the privacy of the individual patient is undermined, effective communication between patients and health care professionals may break down, leading to a situation where patients are unwilling to seek care voluntarily. At the same time third parties may be truly at risk, in which case steps should be taken to facilitate disclosure.

The Government have addressed issues regarding sharing information in the context of mental health in their Draft Bill and consultation on the Mental Health Act 1983 (Department of Health 2002). The Government recognised the tensions between the perceived need for information to ensure effective care and the need to respect the privacy of the individual. They proposed that in relation to the proposed new Mental Health Act there should be a general duty to co-operate in the supply of information regarding risk management and assessment. They also propose that professionals should be subject to a duty to consider as part of the care planning process as to whether there is a duty to share information. It is also envisaged that in relation to bodies which are undertaking functions set out in the new legislation, protocols should be developed supported by a Code of Practice setting out principles (Department of Health 2002 paras 3.27-3.31.) While recognition of the problems in this area and the prospect of structured decision making is to be welcomed, it remains to be seen whether a general duty to co-operate in relation to sharing information regarding risk management and assessment can be seen as something which is in accordance with the Human Rights Act 1998.

Nurses' rights to privacy and confidentiality

Case 5c

> *Jasmin works as a nurse in theatre and has been feeling unwell for some time. She eventually goes to her GP and, based on her symptoms, he suggests that she has a HIV test. The test returns positive. Jasmin needs to work and believes that she is best suited to her current role.*

In such a situation, to what extent can that information be shared within the NHS? Can her GP reveal this information to her employer on the basis that this is in the public interest? Can the information also be used to inform others, such as patients, who may have an interest in knowing whether they themselves may be at risk of infection? In a recent consultation paper (Department of Health 2002) the Department of Health suggested that where health care workers believe that they may have been exposed to HIV infection they should obtain and follow confidential professional advice as to what approach is appropriate, and that to fail to do so would be a breach of duty to the patient (para 4.7). Moreover where health care workers believe that another HIV infected worker is practising in a manner which may put other workers at risk then they must inform the appropriate person in their employing authority (para 4.17). The guidance recognises the need for the confidentiality of HIV positive workers but also that the public interest may in some situations support disclosure but that any such disclosure would require justification (para 10.3) The principle of confidentiality in the context of HIV positive health care workers was confirmed in *X v Y* in 1988 ([1988] 2 All ER 648). But to what extent can it be argued that it is in the public interest to have wider disclosure? What if the press get hold of this information – can they use it as the basis of a newspaper article? In such a situation the media may seek to rely on Article 10 – the right to freedom of expression. Recently the courts have confirmed protection of the confidentiality of health care professionals who are HIV positive, even in a situation in which Article 8 may be seen as in conflict with Article 10 (the right to freedom of expression). In 2002 an injunction was confirmed against The Mail on Sunday preventing disclosure of any information which concerned a NHS healthcare worker (*A (Health Care Worker) v Associated Newspapers Ltd* [2002] EMLR 23). A was HIV positive. He stopped work when he was diagnosed. Department of Health guidelines provided that where patients had undergone procedures where there was a risk of infection then they should be notified that they had been treated by a worker who was HIV positive and they should be offered counselling. The Health Authority wanted to carry out such a look-back study. H was asked to give the Health Authority details of both NHS and private patients. While H returned the details regarding NHS patients because, in his view, the patients were not at risk, he did not return details of the private patients. He brought an action on the basis that the first 'look-back' study was unlawful on the basis of clinical confidentiality. Also he asked for the Health Authority to be restrained from using the information which had been previously supplied. The Mail on Sunday newspaper discovered that this litigation was due to go ahead and wanted to publish details. Their proposed publication of identifying details regarding the clinician and Health Authority was restrained after H brought an action restraining disclosure, which was granted. The paper then brought proceedings seeking to name the Health Authority. At that hearing the Department of Health confirmed that they were intending to introduce guidelines in relation to how look-back studies were to be conducted. On appeal from an interim injunction Gross J held that the Health Authority could be named and that the newspaper could also solicit information regarding the identity of the consultant. On appeal the Court of Appeal considered the argument that this was a newsworthy issue and that no guidelines were currently in existence regarding the notification of patients that they had been treated by a person who was HIV positive. Nonetheless they noted that the paper accepted that H had an interest in his confidentiality and moreover that there was also an interest in preserving the confidentiality of healthcare worker. They were also concerned as to the effects of undue anxiety which could be caused to patients – and indeed it could result in H's identity being revealed through those patients not at risk being informed. The Court of Appeal emphasised the importance of freedom of expression, in particular Article 10, and stated that:

> 'We would view with concern any attempt to invoke the power of the court to restrain an injunction restraining freedom of expression merely on the grounds that release of the information would give rise to administrative problems and a drain on resources. Such consequences are the price which has to be paid for freedom of expression in a democratic society.'

The court emphasised that restraining a newspaper from soliciting information regarding H's area of practice was a draconian fetter on freedom of expression. They also noted the resource issue, namely the cost for the Health Authority in this context of having to be prepared to offer HIV testing and counselling to the patient group treated by clinicians other than in H's patient group – however they were not fully persuaded by this. Here the decisive issue was what would flow from the disclosure of N's identity. The Court of Appeal noted that the possibility of deductive disclosure from disclosure of information regarding N to H's identity was real. However they did not believe that there should be restraint of disclosure of H's specialism.

Interestingly the discussion and emphasis in this case is upon the principle of freedom of expression and its limits rather than that of privacy. In such a situation there are the rights of the health care professional, the rights of freedom of expression of the press and in addition the rights of the public to access the information which may in turn be argued perhaps under Article 8. What this example illustrates fundamentally is the difficult issues which may face a court when in effect having to 'balance' competing rights under the Human Rights Act 1998 in the future.

Rights and genetic information

Case 5d

> *John has been feeling unwell for some time and has now been diagnosed as suffering from Huntington's disease. He is devastated, not just at his own fate but at the implications for his family as the disease is inherited. His brother is soon to be married and has told John that he and his partner hope to have children. John tells the doctor that he does not want anyone to know about the diagnosis.*

Here we again address the question of control of personal information, but in a different way, because what we are dealing with is genetic information. Some regard genetic information as being different or 'special' and that as a consequence the use and control of such information requires specific regulation (see discussion in HGC 2002). It is undoubtedly the case that use of genetic information in a 'family' context can be crucial. Usually people will be willing to share this information amongst their family and extended family. But what if they are not willing? Can the health professional break confidence and disclose? In the case of genetic screening it may be that the boundaries of disclosure of such information have been agreed in advance before the process of screening itself is undertaken. But such agreement has been questioned in the context of genetic screening. It has been suggested that it may be undesirable and indeed may be regarded as coercion to make such agreement a condition of the screening itself being undertaken.

A health professional may break confidence but s/he would need to show that such a breach of confidence was in the public interest. But is it? In the past, disclosure requirements have focused on, for example, matters such as whether harm will be caused. But can harm here be easily detected? It may be the case that disclosure of information may relate to a condition which, if diagnosed, could be cured. In such situations is it a desirable approach to look beyond the principle of individual confidentiality and consider the context of the whole family? In the context of genetic screening and counselling it may be the case that family members have to be involved. The Nuffield Council on Bioethics in their report Genetic Screening noted that in some situations it may be appropriate to regard the family as being a unit (Nuffield 1993). It proposed that where disease would cause grave danger to family members an attempt should be made to ensure that the information was disclosed voluntarily. In exceptional situations information could be disclosed by health professionals to other family members despite an expressed wish for confidentiality if, for example, it was to avoid giving rise to grave damage to family members (Nuffield 1993 para 5.7).

Some commentators suggest that sharing information may be desirable (Skeane 2001). While recognising the importance of confidentiality as a general principle she argues for a family model. First, she suggests, it is the case that genetic conditions generally have a family history and can be family knowledge. Second, clinical experience indicates that individuals are happy to involve families. She distinguishes between two types of genetic information – the first which holds that there is a mutation in the family and the second which relates to the fact that a particular person has tested positive for a condition which is not familial. She also distinguishes between genetic information and genetic material and she says the latter is a biological fact and that this is what blood relatives share.

A difficulty which also arises however is the extent to which the family member to whom the information is disclosed would welcome that information. The unsolicited disclosure of genetic information to relatives will mean that they irreversibly lose their 'genetic innocence' and hence their 'right not to know' (Chadwick 1997). While in a situation in which a condition is curable disclosure may mean that harm is averted this is comparatively rare and few 'cures' exist in relation to genetic conditions (see Laurie 2002 at page 122). As Laurie notes, in a number of studies empirical evidence has been advanced to the effect that knowledge of adverse genetic predispositions may lead to harm – in the case of disclosure of Huntingdon's

Chorea certain studies linked discovery of the diagnosis to an enhanced risk of suicide (in one study Andrews noted that this was at least four times that in the comparable population (Andrews 1990)). The right not to know has also been recognised in certain international rights statements. For example, the Council of Europe Convention for the Protection of Human Rights and Dignity provides that:

> '1. Everyone has the right to respect for private life in relation to information about his or her own health.
>
> 2. Everyone is entitled to know any information collected about his or her own health. However the wishes of individuals not to be so informed shall be observed...'

The Universal Declaration on the Human Genome and Human Rights provides that 'The right of each individual to decide whether or not to be informed of the result of genetic examination and the resulting consequences should be respected'.

A further issue Laurie notes is that of respect. It may be disrespectful, firstly where an individual has expressly stated that she does not wish to know, to furnish the information. Secondly, it may be disrespectful even where there has been no express statement, since to disclose the information will force the person to take on board information and re-evaluate herself. As Laurie states:

> 'It might be argued of course that it is in her best interests to know, but this is to make an evaluative judgment that does not consider the actual wishes of the individual or the full gamut of her interests, including that in not knowing.'

It can thus be argued in a situation in which a condition is incurable such as this that disclosure to the family would not be justifiable and that the individual's privacy should be retained. The genetic correlation of Huntingdon's also would suggest that many family members may be aware of the prospect that they may in any event inherit the condition. However, as noted above, the position regarding other inherited conditions is uncertain. Any decision to disclose would need to be carefully justified by the clinical team on a case-by-case basis. Nurses who work as specialists in the area of genetics and who have ongoing relationships with patient/clients and families are particularly well placed to inform the discussion.

Conclusion

The application of human rights in relation to privacy of personal information has been confirmed by the courts. At the same time Article 8 is, as noted above, a 'qualified right' and thus needs to be weighed against a series of 'public interest' considerations. Furthermore the application of this right may come into conflict with the application of the human rights of other persons – whether Article 2 or Article 8 itself. Respecting the confidentiality and now the privacy of patients has always been problematic. As illustrated above, whilst human rights reasoning may lead us to pause for thought and further consider the boundaries of disclosure it will not provide any easy answers.

There is a further issue, namely the extent to which in the future overt respect for privacy interests may be undermined. One illustration of the ease with which governmental limits may be placed upon the rights of individuals to control access to their personal information arises in the context of Section 60 of the Health and Social Care Act 2001. This Section empowers the Secretary of State to make regulations about disclosing patient information, including mental health information. Regulations may be made that allow information to be processed without a patient's consent (for example, to assist medical research) or prohibit certain disclosures unless consent is first obtained (for example, to stop pharmaceutical companies compiling anonymised information about patients). It effectively grants the Secretary of State power to control information in ways presently forbidden under common law. Although it is a very broad power, there are some limitations. For example, the Secretary of State must consult the Patient Information Advisory Committee established under Section 61 before making any regulations, the use of confidential information must be necessary, regulations must be compatible with the Data Protection Act 1998 and regulations must be reviewed annually to check that they are still necessary. Despite these safeguards, the new regulation making power drew trenchant criticism from the British Medical Association and patient representative groups. The provision was passed without detailed public debate and can be seen as establishing powers that are too wide and unspecified (BMA 2001). The regulations were ultimately passed in Spring 2002. The regulations provide that information can be processed in relation to the diagnosis of communicable disease and other public health risks, the recognition of diseases and risks and controlling their spread, and the monitoring and managing of communicable diseases and incidence of exposure to such disease, delivery and safety of immunisation programmes and adverse reactions to immunisations and medication; it also encompasses disclosure of information relating to diagnosis of communicable diseases and the risks of their acquisition (Health Service (Control of Patient Information) Regulations 2002, SI 2002/1438, reg 4).

While there may indeed a strong arguments to say that the public interest overrides the rights of the individual regarding informational privacy we should surely be circumspect in their use.

References

Andrews L 1990 Legal aspects of genetic information. Yale Journal of Biology and Medicine 64: 29

Beauchamp T L, Childress J F 2001 Principles of biomedical ethics. Oxford University Press, Oxford

Beyleveld D, Histed 2000 Betrayal of confidence in the Court of Appeal. Medical Law International 4: 277

BMA 2001 BMA warns that patient consent and confidentiality are threatened by the Health and Social Care Bill. BMA Press Centre, London

Caldicott 1997 Report on the review of patient identifiable information http://www.doh.gov.uk/confiden.crep.htm

Chadwick R 1997 Genetic screening: Ethical and philosophical perspectives Euroscreen

Counsel and Care 1991 Not such private places. Counsel and Care, London

Department of Health 2000 Consultation on draft mental health bill. http://www.doh.gov/mentalhealth/draftbill2002/consdoc.htm

Department of Health 2002 National service framework for older People. HMSO, London

Department of Health 2002 Health care workers: a consultation paper on management and patient notification. Department of Health, London

Dworkin G 1988 The theory and practice of autonomy. Cambridge University Press, New York

Elliot J 2002 Say goodbye to privacy. The Sunday Times 16/06/02

Gillon 1994 Principles of health care ethics. John Wiley & Sons, Chichester

Gillon 1995 Philosophical medical ethics. BMJ Publishing, Newcastle

Health Advisory Service 2000 Not because they are old – an independent inquiry into the care of older people on acute wards in general hospitals. HAS, London

Human Genetics Commission 2002 Inside information

Kennedy I, Grubb A 2000 Medical law. Oxford Univeristy Press, Oxford

Laurie G 2002 Genetic privacy. Cambridge University Press, Cambridge

Mason J K 2000 The legal aspects and implications of risk assessment. Medical Law Review 8: 69

Montgomery J 2002 Health care law, 2nd edn. Oxford University Press, Oxford

Ngwena C, Chadwick R 1994 Confidentiality and nursing practice: Ethics and law. Nursing Ethics 1 (3): 136-150

NHS Executive 1999 Protecting and using personal information: A manual for Caldicott Guardians

NMC 2002 Code of professional conduct. Nursing & Midwifery Council, London

Nuffield Council on Bioethics 1993 Genetic screening. Butterworths, London

Skeane L 2001 Genetic secrets and the family: A response to Bell and Bennett. Medical Law Review 9: 162

Stone D 2002 Confidentiality, access to health records and the Human Rights Act 1998. In: Garwood-Gowers A, Tingle J Healthcare law: The impact of the Human Rights Act 1998. Cavendish, London

Warren S D, Brandeis L D 1890-91 The right to privacy. Harv LR 193

Woogara J 2001 Human rights and patients' privacy in UK hospitals. Nursing Ethics 8 (3): 234-245

Chapter 6

Rights and allocation of health care resources

Introduction

Nurses play a number of roles in relation to resource allocation in health care. As practitioners with general and specialist skills and knowledge, nurses <u>are</u> a key health care resource. Nurses are also in a position to evaluate existing resources and to raise concerns and highlight inadequacies in care. They can also facilitate patient self-advocacy, or act as advocates on behalf of patients/clients and groups when necessary. In some areas, senior nurses already manage community health budgets. In a recent announcement the Health Secretary, Alan Milburn, promised that ward sisters and charge nurses would gain greater control over wards' staffing budgets (Scott 2001). A number of the ten key roles for nurses outlined in the NHS Plan (Department of Health 2001b) require nurses to make referrals, order diagnostic investigations, prescribe medicines and treatments and to triage patients using information technology. All of these roles have resource implications.

The NMC Code of Professional Conduct (2002) refers explicitly to resources as follows:

'2.1 You must recognise and respect the role of patients and clients as partners in their care and the contributions they can make to it. This involves identifying their preferences regarding care and respecting these within the limits of professional practice, existing legislation, **resources** [our emphasis] and the goals of the therapeutic relationship' (p.3)

Here resources are identified as a limit in relation to patient/client preferences. In Section 1.4 of the NMC Code the duty of care of nurses to patients and clients and their 'entitlement to safe and competent care' is highlighted. Section 8.3 of the NMC Code (2002) states:

'Where you cannot remedy circumstances in the environment of care that could jeopardise standards of practice, you must report them to a senior person with sufficient authority to manage them and also, in the case of midwifery, to the supervisor of midwives. This must be supported by a written record.'

Nurses are obliged to report circumstances which compromise standards of practice. It is possible that inadequate resources, whether human or environmental, may contribute to or be responsible for poor practice. The 1996 (then UKCC) Guidelines for Professional Practice refers explicitly to resources. It states:

'Employers have a duty to provide the **resources** needed for patient and client care, but the numerous requests to the UKCC for advice on this subject indicate that the environment in which care is provided is not always adequate. You may find yourself unable to provide good care because of a lack of adequate resources. Also, you may be afraid to speak out for fear of losing your job. However, if you do not report your concerns, you may be in breach of the Code of Professional Conduct...' (UKCC 1996 p.21)

The UKCC made it clear that nurses are required to report situations when inadequate resources impact negatively on care, regardless of the consequences for the nurse. Employers have a duty to provide the necessary resources. Nurses are required to fulfil their duty of care, to deliver safe and competent care and to respect patients'/clients' preferences but within the limits of resources. Should nurses then accept that patients'/clients' choice may be constrained when resources are inadequate? Which patient/client decisions must be respected regardless of resources? What counts as a fair or just allocation of resources? There is much literature on questions of fairness and justice in relation to resource allocation in health care but no consensus on these matters (see, for example, Gillon 1985 pp.87-8; Doyal 1998, Beauchamp & Childress 2001 Chapter 6; Shickle in Chadwick & Levitt 1998).

So what do patients have a right to regarding health care resources? As discussed in Chapter 1, patients'/clients' rights to health do not extend to everything possible to keep them healthy. As pointed out, many of the contributory factors to health are beyond the scope of health care – factors such as genetic inheritance, lifestyle and the environment, for example. It is arguable that there has been a shift from a focus solely on patients' rights and expectations (as in the 'Patient's Charter') to a view, in its replacement document, 'A Patient's Guide to the NHS' (Department of Health 2001a p.3), which emphasises patients'/clients' responsibilities to promote their own health. 'The NHS Plan' (Department of Health 2001b) states that the first 'core' principle of the NHS is:

> '1. The NHS will provide a universal service for all based on clinical need, not ability to pay. Healthcare is a basic human right.'

'The NHS Plan' also acknowledges that there continues to be inequalities in health, with those in greatest need 'least likely to receive the health services that they require' (the 'inverse care law' – see p.107 'NHS Plan' 2001). Geography is also a factor to be considered in the allocation of resources.

Although the right to health is not explicit in the HRA 1998, Articles 2, 3 and 14 are particularly relevant here. What then are the limits of, for example, Articles 2 (right to life) and 3 (prohibition of torture) regarding resource allocation? Also what impact might Article 14 (prohibition of discrimination) make when policies are in place to limit treatments to those of a certain age? What might ensue when patients/clients and/or staff make resource claims based on requirements of privacy (Article 8) and on their religious or cultural beliefs (Articles 9 and 10)? Finally, what of nurses' rights regarding resource allocation in health care? It is the case that nurses and other professionals are put under additional pressure to deliver quality care when resources are inadequate. Such challenges to professional standards may lead nurses to appeal to Articles 9 (freedom of thought, conscience and religion) and 10 (freedom of expression). Before discussing some of the practical implications of rights in relation to resources, we discuss some of the background to resource allocation in health care.

There has been much debate in recent years about health care resources and the manner in which they are allocated. It has been said that:

> 'No society can afford to offer all its members all the health care that might possibly do them some good. Each society has therefore to establish priorities, it has to decide who will get what and, by implication, who will have to go without.' (Williams in Gillon 1994 p.830)

There is general agreement that scarcity is inevitable in all spheres of life. The slogan 'infinite demand and finite resources' is often presented to capture the present situation in health care. Media reports and journal articles suggest that there are insufficient resources (for example, staff and hospital beds) in the NHS to meet current demands. It has been pointed out that 'although demand may not be infinite, it inevitably reaches boundaries at which the cost of treatment begins to outweigh the benefits, and there may be little consensus about where these boundaries should be' (BMA 2001 p.2). In response to the BMA review the then General Secretary of the Royal College of Nursing, Christine Hancock, said that rationing was a 'policy of despair we are not prepared to adopt' (Parish 2001). In any case, decisions then have to be made about the just allocation of resources – decisions, as Williams suggests above, about who gets what and who will have to go without.

When the NHS was created in 1948 there was optimism that the need for health care spending would decrease as the 'giant of sickness' was conquered (Reid 1998 p.106; New & Le Grand 1996 p.5). However, it has become clear that there has been an increase rather than a decrease in claims on health care expenditure. Common reasons presented for this include demographic changes (most significantly, an increased older population); research and technological developments (for example, developments in genetics and reproductive technologies); and increased expectations. Whilst it has been suggested that there always has been 'implicit rationing' in the NHS via waiting lists and the decisions of doctors, a new management ethos plus demands for evidence-based practice and an increased public awareness has made discussions of resource allocation more public and explicit (Reid 1998 p.106). Developments such as the creation of the National Institute for Clinical Excellence (NICE) in April 1999 might be said to go some way towards ensuring that practice is evidence-based and cost-effective. NICE has the stated role of providing patients, professionals and the public with authoritative, robust and reliable guidance on current 'best practice' (see http://www.nice.org.uk) and would appear to have a role to play in facilitating evidence-based decision-making about the allocation of resources.

Although the focus of this chapter is on rights and resources, it must be said that much discussion of resources is based on utilitarian principles. Cost-benefit analyses of health care interventions are evident in approaches such as QALYs (see Doyal 1998; Edgar in Chadwick 1998). QALYs (quality adjusted life years) have been described as a 'management tool' (Sayers & Nesbitt 2002), designed to estimate which health care treatments or interventions are most efficient, based on cost in relation to benefit which is estimated in terms of expected good quality of life years. The approach has been criticised for being discriminatory (ibid p.9). Older people, for example, have fewer expected life years to live and will therefore do less well when competing for more expensive treatments. Consequentialist or utilitarian arguments in relation to resources allocation are most common, and direct that resources should be allocated in such a way as to maximise utility – that is, in a manner which brings about most benefit to most people. On this view, expensive treatments which benefit only a few people would have a lesser priority.

Around the world, there is concern regarding growing health care costs and about inadequate and inequitable access to services. Different approaches have been taken to resource allocation in health care; some approaches have been incorporated into legislation and others presented as government policy. In 1991 in Oregon in the United States, a state law was passed to expand the Medicaid programme to all those whose income fell below the federal poverty level. However, the Medicaid provision was restricted to health care which appeared on a prioritised list. The Oregon plan, which involved a large consultation exercise, went into effect in February 1994 and an additional 115,000 people became eligible for Medicaid in Oregon. Early reports suggest that the system reduced health care usage in the state (Shickle in Chadwick 1998).

In The Netherlands in 1990 a government committee on choices in health care agreed that 'choices in health care are unavoidable and necessary' and advised that the basic package of mandatory health insurance should contain only care that meets four criteria. It must be: necessary, effective, efficient and cannot be left to the individual's responsibility. The accountability of health professionals was emphasised in assessing effectiveness and appropriateness of care in each case. Treatment choices would be made in the context of health professional standards and guidelines and the committee recommended to the Dutch government that extensive public discussion should occur regarding health choices. Recent judgements of the European Court of Justice (ECJ, *Kohll*, C-158/96 (1998) ECR I-1931; ECJ, *Decker*, C-120/95 (1998) ECR I-1831; *BSM Geraets Smits v Stitching Ziekenfonds VGZ*; *HTM Peerbooms v Stiching CZ Groep Zorgverzekeringen* (2001) Case C-157/99) have made significant developments in relation to European health care by increasing patient choice in obtaining non-emergency healthcare in another European state at the expense of their home state. Some UK NHS hospitals have also arranged for patients to travel to France for treatment (McHale & Bell 2002).

The allocation of resources in health care takes place at three levels. *Micro-allocation* describes allocation which involves decisions amongst individuals; for example, the allocation of intensive care beds, organs or treatments. Nurses in practice will be aware that there are often conflicting demands on their skills and time in relation to individual patients/clients and of the need to allocate their expertise fairly. *Meso-allocation* relates to the allocation of the budget designated for health. Decisions have to be made about the proportion which goes to health providers and specialties. The higher priority, in funding terms, given to acute services over family health services has been questioned (Shickle in Chadwick & Levitt 1998). In a managerial and professional capacity nurses have a role in decision-making at the meso- and micro-allocation levels. Nurses and nursing bodies/unions also assume a political role in influencing decisions about allocation. *Macro-allocation* occurs at a governmental level where decisions are made about the division of the national budget. Health is but one of the social goods which lay claim to the national budget. Spending in other areas, for example, education and housing, will also impact on health. As pointed out in the 'NHS Plan' (2001) referred to above, it is the case that inequalities in health persist and the government has recently outlined targets to end what Deputy Prime Minister, John Prescott, called 'postcode poverty' (Wintour 2001).

In other chapters, issues of rights and resource allocation have been discussed. In Chapter 2, for example, the issue of access to fertility treatment was explored. Here we discuss other issues which have much relevance to resources, rights and nursing practice – namely, the allocation of health care resources in relation to the right to life; in relation to standards of care for older people; and in relation to the allocation of organs.

Resources and the right to life

Case 6a

> *Charlotte, who is seven, has leukaemia and a number of painful treatments have been tried unsuccessfully. The consensus of the team is that treatment should be discontinued as it is not in Charlotte's 'best interests' to continue because the chances of success are remote and that in addition this treatment is very expensive. One team member has suggested that resources should be directed to palliative care. Charlotte's named nurse, Joe, discusses the situation with the parents and finds that Charlotte's parents are adamant that treatment should continue. At the suggestion that treatment cease, the parents become angry and say that Charlotte has a 'right to life'.*

Prior to the HRA 1998 the courts demonstrated, in a series of cases, that they have been unwilling to overturn decisions made by health professionals/managers concerning the allocation of health care resources (Brazier 1993). Since the HRA 1998 came into effect, there have been no challenges thus far on the basis of a right to health care resources. As has been discussed in Chapter 1 the right to health is not absolute, nor is the right to health care unconditional. In England the duties of the Secretary of State for Health regarding the provision of health care are set out in Section 1 of the National Health Service Act 1977, which states:

'It is the Secretary of State's duty to continue the promotion in England and Wales of a comprehensive health service designed to ensure improvement:

a) in the physical and mental health of the people of those countries and

b) in the prevention, diagnosis and treatment of illness

and for that purpose to provide or secure effective provision of services in accordance with the Act.'

Section 3 of that Act states:

'It is the Secretary of State's duty to provide throughout England and Wales to such extent as he considers necessary to meet all reasonable requirements – (a) hospital accommodation... (c) medical, dental, nursing and ambulance services... (f) such other services as are required for the diagnosis and treatment of illness.'

Can the Secretary of State be held liable if services are not provided? In a number of cases persons have challenged a failure to provide health care services in the courts through judicial review proceedings challenging the legality of the decision being made. (Judicial review proceedings enable the court to review a decision on the basis of illegality, irrationality or whether the decision has been reached contrary to the rules of natural justice.) For example, patients in Birmingham challenged the Health Authority's refusal to provide a unit for orthopaedic services (*R v Secretary of State for Social Service ex parte Hincks* [1980] [1979] 123 Sol J 436). The application failed. In the Court of Appeal, Lord Denning ruled that the Secretary of State's duty under the National Health Service Act 1977 needed to be read in the light of the financial resources which he had available. In a later case concerning a similar challenge of failure to provide resources, Stephen Brown LJ stated that:

> 'this is a hearing before a court. This is not the forum in which a court can properly express opinions upon the way in which national resources are allocated or distributed. [There] may be very good reasons why the resources in this case do not allow all the beds in the hospital to be used at this particular time. We have no evidence of that and indeed... it is not for this court or for any other court to substitute its own judgment for the judgement of those who are responsible for the allocation of resources.' (*R v Central Birmingham HA ex parte Collier* [1988] LEXIS 6 January)

This judicial 'hands-off' approach was highlighted in the well-known Child B case. In *ex parte B* Jaymee Bowen ('Child B'), aged 10, developed acute myeloid leukaemia and had treatment which included a bone marrow transplant. After a period of remission the cancer recurred and it was decided by clinicians that no further treatment was appropriate as the chances of a successful outcome were slim. It was also felt that further treatment would be painful and distressing. Jaymee's father sought advice from the United States which suggested that further treatment and a second transplant offered 'a significant chance of success' (New & le Grand 1996 p.7). He challenged Cambridge and Huntington Health Authority in the courts (*R v Cambridge District Health Authority ex parte B* [1995] 2 All ER 129) when they refused to authorise further treatment.

At first instance in the High Court, Laws J said that in determining whether to give treatment, the Health Authority must act reasonably and in making the decision, it should have regard to all relevant considerations. In this case he said the Health Authority had not taken into consideration the views of B's family. He commented that in a situation where, as here, a patient was at risk of death, the Health Authority had to explain why it had decided not to fund the treatment. However, his judgment was overturned in the Court of Appeal. Sir Thomas Bingham MR held that, although the Finance Director of the Health Authority had not spoken directly to the family, he had noted the family's interests. He stated:

> 'Difficult and agonising judgements had to be made as to how a limited budget could best be allocated for the maximum advantage of the maximum number of patients. That was not a judgment for the court.'

Sir Thomas Bingham MR held that in reaching their decision the Health Authority had weighed up the various factors and had not acted unreasonably. Relevant factors were that the treatment was untested and that it could almost be regarded as being experimental in its nature. There was only around a 1-4% success rate. In addition, the court noted the fact that there were potentially debilitating side effects. Overall, it was decided, the decision of the Health Authority was not unreasonable. Ultimately an anonymous donor paid for Jaymee's treatment (donor lymphocyte infusion) and the treatment resulted in remission for over a year. Her cancer returned, however, and Jaymee died in May 1996.

As Brazier has argued:

'the duties to provide health care imposed by Sections 1 and 3 of the 1977 Act are primarily *collective* not individual rights. The individual has no legally enforceable right to demand priority treatment and the courts will intervene to protect the individual interest in the collective right only in the most exceptional and restricted circumstances.' (Brazier 1993)

The Child B case was decided prior to the HRA 1998 (Sullivan 1997). The European Convention on Human Rights and the derivative Human Rights Act 1998, does not make a right to health care resources explicit but it might be argued that the right to life (Article 2) includes a right to health care (ibid p.53). Article 2 states:

'Everyone's right to life shall be protected by law. No one shall be deprived of his life intentionally save in the execution of a sentence of a court following his conviction of a crime for which this penalty is provided by law.'

In the Child B case above, Laws J commented that:

'Of all human rights, most people would accord the most precious place to the right to life itself... If the necessary funds are made available for Dr Gravett to embark on B's treatment, she would enjoy what I would call a worthwhile chance of life. It may be very modest. It may be less than 10%. But to anyone confronting the prospect of extinction in a few weeks, such a chance of longer, perhaps much longer, survival must be unimaginably precious.'

Here, it seems that Laws J equates the right to life with the right to have it prolonged if resources are available, even if the chance of survival is slim. What does this right to life involve? Does it imply a right to have a life of any quality preserved at any cost?

In the Child B case it was argued by Laws J that the right to life would justify embarking on a course of treatment even if the 'chance of life' was 'very modest'. On appeal, however, Sir Thomas Bingham ruled that this was 'not a judgment for the court' but for the Health Authority and that they had weighed up 'the various factors and not acted unreasonably'. He went on to highlight the experimental nature of the treatment and the low chance of success. A distinction has been made between the risk:benefit ratio in this case and the issue of resources.

Following the Child B case, as Outhwaite (2002) notes, the courts have indicated that the allocation of resources by public bodies will be scrutinised by the courts. Nonetheless it is still the case that successful challenges in relation to allocation of NHS resources have been rare. In *R v North Derbyshire HA ex parte Fisher* [1977] 8 Med LR 327 the applicant was refused supply of the drug beta interferon on the basis of advice in a Health Authority policy. The policy allowed the drug to be supplied only where this was in relation to a national clinical trial. The particular difficulty in this situation was that no trials were planned. The Health Authority's policy was itself inconsistent with an NHS Circular, which permitted the introduction of the drug into the system. The Health Authority's decision was struck down. Dyson J held that:

'[T]he policy was unlawful because it was not a proper application of the guidance, contained in the Circular, and the respondents did not properly take into account the essential requirements of the Circular in adopting and maintaining their policy... [The respondents] knew that their own policy amounted to a blanket ban on beta-interferon treatment.'

In *R v Secretary of State for Health ex parte Pfizer Ltd* [1999] Lloyds Rep Med 289, a circular was issued by the Secretary of State with the aim of limiting prescription of Viagra by general practitioners. At that time the NHS terms of service stated that

'a doctor shall order any drugs or appliances which are needed for the treatment of any patient to whom he is providing treatment under these terms of service by issuing to that patient a prescription form.'

The action succeeded as it was held that the doctor was entitled to give such treatment as was considered necessary and appropriate. There is also the prospect for a challenge where resources have been allocated on a basis which is manifestly discriminatory (*R v St Mary's Hospital NHS Trust ex parte Harriot* [1988] 1 FLR 512) (see also Chapter 2 where these issues are the subject of further extensive discussion). More recently in *R v North and East Devon HA ex parte Coughlan* [2000] 2 WLR 622 the decision of a Health Authority to close a residential home for the disabled was overturned in the Court of Appeal. They followed the approach taken in the earlier case of *R v Ministry of Defence ex parte Smith* [1996] QB 517 at p.554 where Sir Thomas Bingham MR stated that:

'The more substantial the interference with human rights, the more the court will require by way of justification before it is satisfied that the decision is reasonable.'

Nonetheless it is uncertain to what extent Charlotte's parents would be successful in the courts in arguing for further treatment on the basis of 'a right to life', particularly as the chances of success here are limited. While the courts have steered away from involvement in many of these cases there is a question as to whether they would ever, as a matter of policy, be prepared to sanction treatment in opposition to a clinically expressed view that treatment was not in a person's best interests. In *Re J (a minor)(consent to medical treatment)* [1992] 4 All ER 614, in a case which concerned the decision whether to ventilate an infant with severe mental disability, cerebral palsy, blindness and epilepsy, Lord Donaldson rejected the notion that the courts could compel clinicians to treat a patient where they are of the view that continued treatment is not in that patient's best interests. However, in a later case, *R v Portsmouth Hospitals NHS Trust ex parte Glass* [1999] LRM 367, Lord Woolf indicated *obitur* that there may be some limited situations in which the courts might be prepared to intervene in the child's best interests. These issues are discussed further in Chapter 8 below.

It has been pointed out that:

> 'It is unclear how far the courts may allow refusal of life-saving treatment to be raised under Article 2 in individual cases, though medical authorities may need to justify their general policies on the use of medical resources.' (Home Office 2000 p.10)

Some suggestions have been made under the ECHR that there may be a positive obligation upon the state to protect life. For example in *LCB v UK* (1998) 27 EHRR 212 it was stated that:

> 'The first sentence of Art 2(1) enjoins the state not only to refrain from the intentional and unlawful taking of life but also to take appropriate steps to safeguard the lives of those within its jurisdiction.'

Similarly in *Osman v UK* (1999) 29 EHRR 245, a wider positive duty to save life was also recognised. However the English courts have been circumspect in interpreting the Convention. The right to life in the context of the minor or mentally incompetent adult is considered in the light of what clinical procedures are in their best interests (e.g. *A NHS Trust v D* [2000] TLR 552) and this issue is discussed further in Chapter 8. It may be the case that a different approach will be taken if the sole reason for refusing the therapy was that of lack of resources. In *Scialacqua v Italy* (1998) 26 EHRRS 164 the Commission took the view that Article 2 did impose an obligation to meet costs of life-saving therapy (Outhwaite 2002). Nonetheless in *Osman v UK* (2000) 29 EHRR 245 the European Court of Human Rights held that Article 2:

> 'must be interpreted in a way which does not impose an impossible or disproportionate burden on the authorities. Accordingly not every claimed risk to life can entail for the authorities a Convention requirement to take operational measures to prevent that risk from materialising.'

There is a possibility that other rights, such as Article 3 (freedom from torture, inhuman or degrading treatment) might be brought in to counter the right to life in a situation such as that of Charlotte. Should further treatment be considered painful or too burdensome, Article 3 might apply as further therapy may not be regarded as being in the patient's best interests. However, application of Article 3 may also support Charlotte's parents' claims. In *Tanko v Finland* (Case 23634/94 (1994) unreported) it was held that to fail to provide 'proper medical treatment' can contravene Article 3. A further issue is whether Article 8 may be applicable in such a situation. Maclean (2002) notes that one argument which can be advanced is that as health can be seen as a moral value from an individual and from a social perspective, and an individual choice as to what amounts to health should be respected by the state. The prospect of whether Articles 3 and 8 can be used in a case where funding for treatment is sought was raised in relation to a case where there was a successful challenge to a Health Authority's general policy to refuse to fund gender reassignment surgery for transsexuals (*R v North West Lancashire HA v A* [2000] 2 FCR 525 CA). Auld J commented that Article 3 was not designed for circumstances of the sort where the challenge was to a health authority's allocation of finite funds between competing demands. Auld J also commented that the notion of 'respect' for private and family life under Article 8 was not clear-cut. He stated that:

> 'In determining whether or not a positive obligation exists, regard must be had to the fair balance that has to be struck between the general interests of the community and the interests of the individual, the search for which balance is inherent in the whole Convention.'

The nurse, Joe, in the case study is caring for the family although his priority is the welfare and well-being of Charlotte. This scenario raises a potential rights conflict – that of Charlotte's rights and 'best interests' and parental rights. When faced with a choice between certain death and even a slim chance of survival, it is understandable why parents might choose the latter. Charlotte is seven years old and it is not stated what she knows or understands about her condition or treatment/care options. No doubt adults will wish to protect her from further suffering but it may be that she is not being heard. The mother of a seriously ill child (cited by Alderson 1990 p.222) wrote:

> 'We should look at what the child's behaviour is telling us. Remembering the difficulty I, as an adult, had in being heard, I am confident that many children suffer from being unheard. Especially because so much of what they have to tell us is said non-verbally. People should ask themselves if they are really 'listening' in every sense of that word.'

This raises the question of whether adults have a right to make difficult treatment decisions without informing younger patients. Article 12 of the UN Convention on the Rights of the Child (1989) supports the right of the child to be heard in 'in any judicial and administrative proceedings affecting the child, either directly, or through a representative or an appropriate body, in a manner consistent with the procedural rules of national law'. Nurses have an important advocacy role to play in cases such as Child B and the case of Charlotte. They may enable parents to consider all relevant information about treatment/care options and to 'listen' to the child. Nurse specialists are also in an important role to provide explanations about established and experimental treatments and palliative care options, and to counsel families when difficult decisions have to be made. The impact of the Patient Advocacy and Liaison Services (PALS) outlined in the 'NHS Plan' (2001b) has yet to be felt but may be instrumental in supporting patients in resource decisions.

Resources and standards of care: blowing the whistle

Case 6b

> *Christine is a registered nurse and works on an Accident and Emergency department. The department is frequently short-staffed and often there are not enough beds in the hospital for patients who have been treated. It is not uncommon for elderly patients to remain on trolleys for long periods. It is sometimes difficult to spend sufficient time with patients to provide reassurance and assistance. The environment is shabby and there are, on a regular basis, inadequate gowns for patients and a shortage of linen. Occasionally, patients/clients have to make do with pillow cases when there are no more towels. Christine has complained to her ward manager on many occasions but his response is that they have to 'make do' as 'every area in the hospital is in the same position'.*

In August 1989 Graham Pink, a night charge nurse on the care of the elderly wards at Stepping Hill Hospital, Stockport, wrote to Stockport Health Authority about his concerns about the welfare of patients. The neglect he detailed was attributed to staff shortages. In April 1990, after writing some fifty letters, Mr Pink allowed a section of his letters to be published in The Guardian newspaper. Mr Pink was advised not to speak out further. During one of the night shifts in July 1990, an 82-year-old patient on Mr Pink's ward called out for a bottle. As Mr Pink was attending to another patient he could not respond and he later found the patient lying on the floor sobbing, in a pool of urine. Mr Pink told the Editor of the Stockport Express about the incident. In August 1990, Mr Pink was suspended from duty – charges against him included breach of confidentiality. A subsequent industrial tribunal action which he brought was settled (McHale 1992).

In the Pink case, inadequate staffing levels and subsequent lack of appropriate care for a highly dependent group of older patients led to his whistleblowing. Whilst this case occurred over a decade ago, there continues to be concern about staffing levels and about the treatment of older people in hospital. The Health Advisory Service 2000 'Not because they are old' inquiry into the care of older people on acute wards, for example, pointed to deficiencies in the physical environment, staff shortages, lack of time, the non-availability and poor quality of food and drink and to problems with the maintenance of dignity and individuality (HAS 1998). Research studies have also suggested age discrimination in relation to the management of trauma, staff attitudes, and the availability of palliative care for older people (see Department of Health 2001c National Service Framework for Older People p.16-17; Health Advisory Service 2000; Sayers & Nesbitt 2002). There has also been concern expressed about the allocation of life-saving procedures and transplants to older patients. A recent survey of managers in the NHS and social care found that 'three out of four senior managers believed age discrimination existed in their local services, and many felt that ageism was endemic' (Roberts & Seymour 2002).

In the Pink case there was a discrepancy between what the Health Authority and Mr Pink viewed as 'adequate care'. The Health Authority prepared a report on staffing levels at Stepping Hill Hospital, using a method which listed six levels of care – dangerous, barely safe, less than adequate, adequate, good and excellent. The Health Authority report concluded that 'standards of care were adequate, given the level of resources' (Turner 1992 p.28). It did conclude that in one of the wards standards were not always adequate. Nurses may indeed believe that they are better placed to determine adequate standards of care due to their close contact with patients/clients. Pink writes:

> 'We, the nurses, are there at the bedside, day and night. As no one else is. We are better placed to ensure that the care that the NHS provides meets patients' needs and expectations and does so to an acceptable professional standard. But we are being silenced by evasive, gutless managers and undemocratic structures. These structures stifle public debate about staffing levels and standards of care.' (Pink 1994 p.1704)

The case of Graham Pink undoubtedly raises key questions about freedom of expression and privacy or confidentiality (Articles 8 and 10 of the HRA 1998). Some of these issues have been discussed the previous chapter. Whilst there is an imperative for nurses to report poor practice, utilising the HRA 1998 to defend patients' rights may be practically problematic. One possibility is that patients may bring an action before the courts on the basis that resources are inadequate. In the past while there has been the prospect that there may be liability in civil law in the form of an action in negligence if resources are inadequate, such an action would be problematic (Brazier 1993). Although an action may potentially be brought under the tort of breach of statutory duty (in this case, the infringement of the obligations of the Secretary of State under the NHS Act 1977) in practice this would be difficult as the English courts have been reluctant to take such an approach and extend liability in such a situation (e.g. *R v Secretary of State for Social Services ex parte Hincks* [1980] BMLR 93). Nonetheless once treatment has begun there is the possibility that an action in negligence may be brought on the basis that there has been inadequate organisation of health care based on the direct liability of the NHS body (*Robertson v Nottingham HA* [1997] 8

Med LR 1). Such an action may potentially be rooted in a claim that the provision of resources was inadequate (*Re HIV Haemophiliac Litigation* [1996] PIQR P220 and see Lee 2002). Today such actions may also be bolstered by the provisions of the Human Rights Act.

Patients/clients may bring a case to the British courts against the Health Authority on the basis of Articles 2, 3 and/or 14 if they believe their rights to life, dignity and fair treatment have been compromised. It has been suggested that Article 2 (right to life) may be interpreted more broadly than 'refrain from taking life' and should include taking 'appropriate steps to safeguard life' (Sayers & Nesbitt 2002 p.12). Further:

'This has been taken to mean that in addition to the requirement of 'reasonable care' imposed by ordinary domestic law of negligence, the advent of the Human Rights Act will require doctors and NHS Trusts to provide adequate care or appropriate levels of healthcare.' (ibid p.12)

In the light of comments from the European Commission, it is suggested that Article 2 could impose on states the 'obligation to cover the costs of medical treatment essential to life' (ibid).

The example above of an older patient lying in his own urine raises the issue of dignity which appears as a central concept in international rights declarations such as the Universal Declaration of Human Rights. The preamble states:

'Whereas recognition of the inherent dignity and of the equal and inalienable rights of all members of the human family is the foundation of freedom, justice and peace in the world...'

Dignity also appears as a professional value in the NMC Code of Professional Conduct (2002). Section 2.2 states:

'You are personally accountable for ensuring that you promote and protect the interests and dignity of patients and clients...'

Although dignity is not made explicit in the Human Rights Act 1998, it can be argued that it appears negatively as Article 3:

'No one shall be subjected to torture or to inhuman or degrading treatment or punishment.'

In *Tanko v Finland* (Case 23634/94 (1994)) the European Court of Human Rights held that failing to provide 'proper medical treatment' may constitute an infringement of Article 3.

A recent pilot study by Seedhouse and Gallagher (2002) highlighted resources (sufficient staff, equipment and linen) as a factor which promoted or diminished dignity in practice.

Since the Pink affair there have been some further developments which would now impact in such a situation. As stated in the introduction, the NMC requires nurses to report poor standards of practice and resources may be a causative factor here. Whilst there is an obligation or duty to report poor practice, there is no right to whistleblow in the HRA 1998 although nurses may seek to use Article 9 (freedom of thought, conscience and religion) and Article 10 (freedom of expression). There is, however, a potential rights conflict with Article 8 (right to respect for private and family life) should nurses go public with information considered confidential, a tension illustrated by the Pink case itself. These issues are discussed in more detail in Chapter 5. There is now specific legislation which may protect whistleblowers in the form of the Public Interest Disclosure Act 1998. This legislation aims to protect whistleblowers from victimisation and dismissal and may have assisted Christine, in the scenario above, if she decided to take her complaint further and this resulted in adverse consequences for her (McHale & Tingle 2001; Lee 2002). However this is applicable once a person wishes to challenge action taken against them by their employer and bring an action before an employment tribunal. In many respects the provisions of this legislation can be seen as a 'last resort' measure. Where an employee has been dismissed for 'blowing the whistle' by, for example, as in the case of Pink, going to the press, reinstatement is likely to be rare.

Nurses have 24-hour access to the experience of patients/clients. This puts them in a special position to promote patient self-advocacy and, when involved with more vulnerable and incompetent patients/clients, to act as advocates on their behalf. When resources are inadequate, there may be inadequate time or motivation to find out about and respect patient preferences and choices. Lack of resources (particularly staff and equipment) may lead to patients/clients being harmed more than helped by health care. Where resources are scarce vulnerable groups, such as older people and the disabled, may be treated unjustly.

It is uncertain how the courts will determine issues concerning relation to rights, resources and standards of practice and whether and when patients/clients and relatives will resort to the HRA 1998 to attempt to remedy resourcing deficits which impact negatively on everyday practice. There have been high profile cases where patients/clients and/or their families have been unhappy with standards of care in the Accident and Emergency department. Cases such as that of Thomas Rogers, who died in A&E at Whipps Cross Hospital in October 2001 after a nine-hour wait, led to an independent inquiry which reported that staff levels were too low and the workforce 'accepted grossly inadequate outcomes as normal' (Akid 2002).

Clearly inadequate resourcing may compromise standards of care. In the Pink case, and perhaps in the case of Christine above, it seems plausible that increased funding would have led to the employment of more qualified nurses, more linen and an improved environment, thus improving standards of care. Current initiatives such as the National Service Framework for the Care of Older People (Department of Health 2001c) go some way to promoting parity and eliminating discrimination directed at vulnerable groups.

Rights and the allocation of organs

Case 6c

> *Martin is gravely injured in a road traffic accident. He is put into ITU and maintained on life support systems. His relatives are told that he is near death. They are asked to consider whether they will allow his organs to be used for transplantation purposes. His family say yes, but only if the organs go to a Christian recipient. They say that this is also stipulated on Martin's organ donor card. The transplant co-ordinator is shocked by this request and consults her line-manager.*

Organs are a scarce resource and hard decisions have to be made regarding their allocation (New, Solomon, Dingwall & McHale 1994). There is no 'right' to an organ nor is there a right to determine how a donated organ should be allocated. An appeal to the 'right to life' given the scarcity of such a precious resource would be futile. It is likely that nurses who work as transplant co-ordinators would find the case above particularly challenging.

The Human Tissue Act 1969 allows patients to donate organs during their lifetime (Section 1(1)) and it also allows the use of organs after their death in a situation in which there is no express request, for example, through a donor card where 'such inquiries as are reasonably practicable' as to whether the deceased had expressed an objection or that the spouse/surviving relatives had any objection (Section 1(2) Human Tissue Act 1961). The Act itself remains silent upon the issue as to whether any conditions could be placed upon donation. A similar incident which arose in the North West led to a report upon Conditional Organ Donation (Department of Health 2001). This was very critical of the decision to agree to accept organs subject to such conditions.

It should be noted that in the context of the use of tissue from aborted foetuses, the guidelines into the use of foetal tissue issued after the Polkinghorne Committee Report state that while women can give general consent to the use of the material, they cannot state that it must be used for specific purposes (Polkinghorne 1989). While Article 14 of the ECHR does provide for a principle of non-discrimination this provision can only operate in conjunction with other Convention rights and does not by itself establish a scheme of non-discrimination. Although there is explicit legislative provision in England in relation to race, sex and disability discrimination (Race Relations Act 1974; Sex Discrimination Act 1975; Disability Discrimination Act 1995) there is currently no statutory provision made for age discrimination.

Martin's family could argue that Article 8, the right to privacy, encompasses also his right to autonomy in determining how his organs should be allocated. Article 8 may be relevant in relation to Martin's rights which may continue after death. It is uncertain as to whether the ECHR would apply post death in such a situation. Alternatively the family may use

Article 8 on their own account. As Garwood-Gowers (2002) commented:

> 'the notion of family life under Art 8 ought to provide an opportunity for a close relative to take action as a closely associated person who might be classed as a victim in his or her own right if extraction, use or disposal of the deceased's bodily materials is taking place in a manner contrary to rights.'

We return to this issue in the following chapter, where we consider the whole question of use of human material post-Alder Hey. However, it is questionable whether such a right could extend so far as to include conditional donation. If this were permitted, then it is arguable that Health Authorities would be colluding with discriminatory practices, and in the example above, violating the human rights of non-Christian patients who were awaiting organ transplantation. Even if it was argued in such a situation that Martin's organs were 'property' or the property of his family, public policy considerations would undoubtedly operate against conditional donations.

Conclusion

Here we have discussed some of the rights issues which have relevance to resource allocation in health care. In the case of Child B, and cases where individuals have appealed for access to reproductive technologies, the courts have not thus far overturned rulings of NHS bodies regarding resource allocation restrictions. The Pink case raised many issues about the role of nurses in attempting to remedy inadequate care situations due to under-resourcing. Nurses are obliged by the NMC to report poor standards of care. Whilst nurses may claim that they have rights of free speech and freedom of conscience in the HRA 1998, it may be that that legislation such as the Public Interest Disclosure Act 1998 will be more effective in protecting nurses who go public about poor standards. The allocation of organs is a particularly difficult resource issue given that patients/clients are seriously ill and dependent on donation. The Department of Health report on conditional organ donation argued that attaching conditions to organs in donation is unsatisfactory and may, in fact, violate the human rights of others.

Nurses have an important role to play at all levels of resource allocation. The issues discussed in this chapter highlight the nurse's direct involvement in resource allocation decision-making, in promoting patient/client self-advocacy and in speaking out when resources are inadequate. It is uncertain what role the HRA 1998 will play in redressing poor resourcing in the NHS as clients/patients and their families may continue to seek compensation and redress through the civil and criminal courts. It may be that claims to access expensive and innovative treatments will be made in the future but again, it is uncertain whether the judiciary in a human rights culture will be responsive to such challenges.

References

Akid M 2002 Staffing levels too low A & E staff tell trust. Nursing Times 98 (4)

Alderson P 1990 Choosing for children – parents' consent to surgery. Oxford University Press, Oxford

Beauchamp T L, Childress J F 2001 Principles of biomedical ethics, 5th edn. Oxford University Press, Oxford

BMA 2001 Healthcare funding review. British Medical Association, London

Brazier M 1993 Rights and healthcare. In: Blackburn R (ed) Rights of citizenship. Mansell

Department of Health 2001a A patient's guide to the NHS. HMSO, London

Department of Health 2001b NHS Plan – a plan for investment, a plan for reform. HMSO, London

Department of Health 2001c National service framework for older people. HMSO, London

Doyal L 1998 Needs, rights and equity: Moral quality in healthcare rationing. In: Quality in Healthcare 4: 273-283

Edgar A 1998 Quality of life indicators. In: Chadwick R (ed) Encyclopedia of applied ethics, volume 3. Academic Press, San Diego

Garwood-Gowers A 2002 Use of materials for transplantation and research. In: Garwood-Gowers A, Tingle J, Lewis T (eds) Healthcare law: The impact of the Human Rights Act 1998. Cavendish, London

Gillon R 1985 Philosophical medical ethics. John Wiley & Sons, Chichester

Health Advisory Service 2000 Not because they are old – an independent inquiry into the care of older people on acute wards in general hospitals. HAS, London

Home Office 2000 Study guide – Human Rights Act 1998. Home Office Communications Directorate, London

Lee R 2002 Responsibility, liability and scarce resources. In: Cribb A, Tingle J (eds) Nursing law and ethics, 2nd edn. Blackwell Scientific, Oxford

Maclean A 2002 The individual's right to treatment under the Human Rights Act. In: Garwood-Gowers A, Tingle J, Lewis T (eds) Healthcare law: The impact of the Human Rights Act 1998. Cavendish, London

McHale J V 1992 Whistleblowing in the NHS. Journal of Social Welfare Law 5: 363

McHale J, Tingle J 2001 Law and nursing. Butterworth-Heinemann, Oxford

McHale J, Bell M 2002 Travellers checks. Health Service Journal 112: 39

New B, Solomon M, Dingwall R, McHale J 1994 A question of give and take: Increasing the supply of donor organs for transplantation. King's Fund, London

New B, Le Grand J 1997 Rationing in the NHS – Principles and pragmatism. King's Fund, London

NMC 2002 Code of professional conduct. NMC, London

O'Sullivan D 1998 The allocation of scarce resources and the right to life under the European Convention on Human Rights. Public Law 385

Outhwaite W 2002 Impact of the HRA on healthcare and NHS resource allocation. In: Garwood-Gowers A, Tingle J (eds) Healthcare law: The impact of the Human Rights Act 1998. Cavendish, London

Parish C 2001 Nurses and doctors split over need to ration care. Nursing Standard 15 (22): 9

Pink G 1994 The price of truth. British Medical Journal 309: 1700-1705

Polkinghorne J 1989 Review of the guidance on research use of fetuses and fetal material. Cmnd 762. HMSO, London

Reid J 1998 Blanket ban on treatment: Conflict in healthcare resourcing. British Journal of Nursing 7 (2): 105-110

Roberts E, Seymour L 2002 Old habits die hard. King's Fund, London

Sayers G, Nesbitt T 2002 Ageism in the NHS and the Human Rights Act 1998: An ethical and legal inquiry. European Journal of Health Law 5

Scott G 2001 Milburn promises more control over staff budgets. Nursing Standard 16 (10): 4

Seedhouse D, Gallagher A 2002 Undignifying institutions. Journal of Medical Ethics 28 (6): 366

Shickle D 1998 Rationing of health care: why do acute hospital services have high priority? In: Chadwick R, Levitt M (eds) Ethical issues in community healthcare. Arnold, London

Shickle D 1998 Resource allocation. In: Chadwick R (ed) Encyclopedia of applied ethics, volume 3. Academic Press, San Diego

Turner T 1992 The indomitable Mr Pink. Nursing Times 28 (24): 26-29

UKCC 1996 Guidelines for professional practice. United Kingdom Central Council for Nursing, Midwifery and Health Visiting, London

Williams A 1994 Economics, society and health care ethics. In: Gillon R (ed) Principles of health care ethics. John Wiley & Sons, Chichester

Websites

National Institute for Clinical Excellence – http://nice.org.uk

Chapter 7

Research and rights

Introduction

It is only relatively recently that research has come to play a recognised role in nursing. In 1972, for example, the Committee on Nursing emphasised the need to bring 'research-mindedness' into the curriculum and suggested that nursing should become a research-based profession (Kenkre et al 2001). The movement of nurse education from the NHS to higher education institutions has facilitated an enhanced appreciation of research in relation to health and illness. There is now an acknowledged career pathway in research for nurses and whilst some nurses may choose research as a career option, it has been highlighted that 'research is everybody's business and not a discipline to be conducted solely through academic institutions' (ibid p.40).

Nurses play various roles in health care research – as researchers, as research subjects, as members of research ethics committees and as patient advocates when patients/clients in their care are involved in research. Nurses, in the role of research assistants or research nurses, will generally take care of the practical aspects of a study, including data collection and analysis. They will work within a research protocol generally devised by more senior members of the research team. In everyday practice, nurses will care for patients who have been invited to participate, or who are participating in, health care research. The role of nurses as patient advocates is particularly important here as patients are in a vulnerable position and may not be in a position to make an 'informed consent'. The involvement of nurses in clinical research came under recent criticism in the Griffiths Inquiry (NHSE 2001) into the conduct of trials into CNEP (Continuous Negative Extrathoracic

Pressure) on infants at North Staffordshire hospital (Griffiths 2001). The Inquiry found that the nursing sister who was assigned to the project did not appear to have been given a protocol or appropriate documentation and that nursing staff involved in the project were inadequately experienced and had not been given the opportunity of training.

As members of research ethics committees, nurses are involved in the sanctioning of good research and in the vetoing of research which violates the rights of patients and/or others. Nurses may also be approached to participate in research as subjects. Some of this research may be qualitative in nature (a study, for example, which enquires about nurses' views of caring). Nurses and students of nursing may also be recruited as healthy volunteers to participate in medical trials. In all of these roles, it is in the interests of nurses, patients and indeed society as a whole, that nurses have a good grasp of ethical, professional and legal aspects of research.

The NMC Code of Professional Conduct (2002) makes explicit mention of research as follows:

'6.5 You have a responsibility to deliver care based on current evidence, best practice and, where applicable, validated research when it is available.'

However, the Code is as applicable to health care research, where nurses are involved, as to practice. Sections which direct nurses to respect individuality, obtain consent, protect confidential information, maintain professional knowledge and competence, be trustworthy and act to identify and minimise risk, are also important directives for research.

There are many rights issues which relate to research but these have yet to be tested under the HRA 1998. In this chapter, we will explore some of the human rights implications of health care research in the context of existing law and professional guidelines, and point to some specific research areas which may lead to challenges in the future.

Research in its broadest sense involves balancing the rights of individual research subjects (be they patients/clients or healthy volunteers) with the researcher's wish to develop knowledge. As the BMA (2001 p.105) points out:

'The very potential for achieving tangible benefits can feed the temptation to press on beyond acceptable boundaries. Utilitarian arguments about an anticipated greater good are commonly invoked by those willing to sacrifice the rights of research subjects. In addition to humanitarian aims, scientific curiosity is another major impetus for experimentation.'

In research there is much potential for harm and unethical practice. The history of research in relation to health highlights many human rights violations. During World War 2, many atrocities were carried out in the name of 'scientific experimentation' in the concentration camps (BMA 1993 p.204; BMA 2001 Chapter 9). Such 'research' on non-consenting individuals mobilised the international community to draft research codes and declarations with a view to preventing such abuses occurring again. The Nuremberg Code and the World Medical Association Declaration of Helsinki are examples. The Nazi experiments are not the only examples of research abuse in the last century. One of the most notorious illustrations of research abuse was the Tuskeegee experiments conducted in the period 1932-1972. Afro-American men in Alabama, who suffered from syphilis, were given placebos or left untreated even though penicillin was available as an effective treatment (Jones 1981; BMA 2001 p.220). More recently, in 1990, it has been documented that British soldiers who were sent to the Gulf were given 'cocktails of drugs'. Although policies of 'voluntary informed consent' were in place, there was 'strong pressure' to agree (BMA 2001 p.212). Coercion to take part in research violates the individual's autonomy. It has also been argued that 'lack of opportunity' to participate in research can also be abusive. As the BMA (2001 p.208) states:

> 'Since the thalidomide tragedy in the 1960s, a principal concern has been to protect people from the potential hazards of experimental drugs but now in the AIDS era early access to experimental therapies is often viewed as an opportunity or even a benefit to which people are entitled, rather than a burden from which they must be protected. Harm can result from the complete exclusion of some categories of patient, such as children and the elderly, from research that could benefit that group.'

Despite a proliferation of research guidelines, there continues to be evidence of research abuses and fraud. Research in the US in the 1960s highlighted fifty unethical studies and suggested many more (BMA 1997 p.201). In the UK Papworth (1967) also pointed to research abuses. His study was influential in the establishment of ethics committees. The existence of such committees has not, however, eliminated all unethical research. The Lancet detailed a 1981 case of an elderly woman who died from bone marrow depression in the course of a drug trial. The trial had been approved by eleven ethics committees (BMA 1993 p.202). In the 1980s there was much public concern about the deaths of two young medical students who had volunteered to participate in clinical trials of new drugs (BMA 1993 p.201). In 2000, the death of a young woman who had taken part in a trial at Johns Hopkins in the U.S. caused much concern within and without the research community (Keigher & de Pasquale 2002).

Before discussing specific examples, we will discuss what research involves, what legislation exists to regulate health care research and which articles of the HRA 1998 would appear to have most relevance to this area.

Research has been defined variously. Seedhouse (2000 p.79) defines it as:

> 'Any method, applied to any phenomenon, that can produce a greater understanding of that phenomenon.'

On this account a wide range of activities count as research and 'every inquisitive nurse' (ibid) may be considered a researcher. Research has also been defined as:

'the systematic and rigorous process of enquiry which aims to describe phenomena and to develop explanatory concepts and theories. Ultimately it aims to contribute to a scientific body of knowledge.' (Bowling 1997 p.1)

Research on this account is not just about the envisaged goal of enhanced understanding. It is also a process undertaken in a 'systematic and rigorous way'.

Distinctions are made between health research and health services research (Bowling 1997) and also between medical and nursing research. A further distinction is made between therapeutic and non-therapeutic research and innovative treatment (BMA 1993). Therapeutic research can be defined as being research where the aim is diagnosis and therapy for the patient, whereas the objective of non-therapeutic research is to extend knowledge with a view to benefiting future patients. Interestingly the most recent version of the Declaration of Helsinki does not make reference to non-therapeutic research. Although there are indications given that the inclusion of healthy volunteers in research may be ethical, as Forster, Emanuel and Grady (2001) argue:

'Nonetheless the overarching tone of the Declaration and of several specific provisions suggest that benefit to participants is necessary for research to be ethical.'

Innovative treatments are said to straddle research and medical practice. A high profile example might be the treatment of Jaymee Bowen, discussed in Chapter 4, or the case of one-year-old, Laura Davis, who went to the United States for a multi-organ transplant. It is acknowledged that the boundaries between these categories may be blurred and that there may be overlap. Innovative treatments are particularly controversial and have been described as a trial and error approach.

One difficult issue is the interrelationship between innovative therapy and clinical trials. For the first time it appears that there will be a coherent overview, as following the recommendations made by the Kennedy Report following the Bristol Inquiry, the National Institute of Clinical Excellence (NICE) assumed responsibility for the 'Safety and Efficacy Register of Interventional Procedures' (see http://www.nice.org.uk/cat.asp?).

The degree of patient/subject involvement in research varies a great deal. Many medical research studies require participants to take drugs (randomised controlled trials, for example) or to have invasive procedures. Other studies require patients/subjects to donate tissue for analysis. Some studies require patients/subjects to answer questions, to complete questionnaires or to agree to be observed in their patient or professional roles. Some studies require no direct patient involvement – for example, those which involve medical/nursing records.

There is now much discussion of the ethical, legal and professional aspects of research practice. There is no one single piece of legislation which governs all clinical research on human subjects. Thus general common law and statutory principles are applicable as are some specific provisions from, for example, the European Union, as we shall see below (see Fox 2002; McHale & Fox 1997). Research is informed by guidelines produced by the Government, for example, the Department of Health guidelines on research governance and by bodies such as the Medical Research Council and the Association of the British Pharmaceutical Industry.

The health professions have also published guidelines relating to research, some of which make explicit reference to human rights. Probably the most significant professional guidance/directive is the World Medical Association Declaration of Helsinki, now in its fifth revision (http://www.wma.net /e/policy/17-c_e.html). The Declaration states, for example:

'8. Medical research is subject to ethical standards that promote respect for all human beings and protect their health and **rights**...

10. It is the duty of the physician in medical research to **protect the life, health, privacy and dignity of the human subject**...'

The revised Declaration represents an important document. It states that it is a 'statement of ethical principles' and has priority over national laws and regulations. For example Provision 9 now states that 'No national, ethical, legal or regulatory requirement should be allowed to reduce or eliminate any of the protections for human subjects set forth in this Declaration.' However, while the Declaration may claim to offer definitive guidance, it has been noted that 'The authority and practical meaning of this self-proclaimed status is unclear' (Forster, Emanuel & Grady 2001).

The Council of Europe has been active in the production of statements applicable to clinical practice and research, notably the Convention on Human Rights and Biomedicine (1997). This Convention which is discussed in Chapter 1 provides a broad range of statements on rights in relation to the research process. The UK Government is however not currently a signatory to this Convention (Plomer 2001). Chapter V of the Convention focuses explicitly on scientific research. The regulation of clinical trials now needs to be seen in the context of the developments in the EU in the form of the Clinical Trials Directive regarding the conduct of trials on medicinal products (OJ c306, 18:10:97). The Directive provides that clinical trials must be conducted in accordance with good clinical practice guidelines. While this Directive relates to trials undertaken on medicinal products it has been suggested that its impact is one which is capable of extending more broadly (Montgomery 2002).

Concerns regarding potential abuses in clinical research were highlighted in an inquiry into the effectiveness of continuous negative extra-thoracic pressure with standard positive pressure ventilation in some 244 preterm babies. The inquiry followed allegations that parents had been not asked to give adequately informed consent (NHSE 2001). The inquiry was exceedingly critical of the conduct of the trial and we refer to it elsewhere in this chapter. It led the inquiry team to call for a national framework of research governance. In May 2000 the Government accepted the recommendations and Lord Hunt, Health Minister, issued a statement which included a commitment to the development of a framework for research governance (Ramsey 2000). The Research Governance Guidance which was subsequently published states that 'The dignity, rights, safety and well-being of participants must be the primary consideration in any research study' (Department of Health 2001 para 2.2.1). All research which involves patients, service users, care professionals or volunteers or their organs, tissue or data is required to be the subject of independent ethical review. The guidelines emphasise that: 'Research and those pursuing it should respect the diversity of human culture and conditions and take full account of ethnicity, gender disability, age and sexual orientation in its design, undertaking and reporting. Researchers should take account of the multi-cultural nature of society' (para 2.2.7).

The Research Governance Framework states that a quality research culture is essential for proper governance of health and social care research and the Guidelines set out the consitituent parts of this framework as follows:

'Respect for participants' dignity, rights, safety and well being

Valuing the diversity within society

Personal and scientific integrity

Leadership

Honesty

Accountability

Openness.' (para 2.7.2)

It is regarded as good practice to refer all clinical trials to research ethics committees (RECs) for approval. The Department of Health has recently published new guidelines for RECs (Department of Health 2001). Research ethics committees are local committees drawn from backgrounds in clinical, non-clinical, qualitative and other methods of social science research which also includes statistics, clinical practice which includes hospital and community staff including medical, nursing and others (Department of Health 2001 Section 6). The guidance requires that at least one third of the membership should be 'lay'. These are considered further below. Research ethics committees are now co-ordinated by the Central Office for Research Ethics Committees. This body also acts a resource for REC training and advises on policy concerning research ethics (http://www.corec.org.uk). In the case of research involving five or more REC centres then an application must be made to a multi-centre research ethics committee. Ethics are regarded as being one part of clinical research governance standards (Department of Health 2001).

The HRA 1998 has still to be tested in relation to health research and it is possible the following Articles will have a bearing on research in health care:

- Article 2 (right to life) – This Article may be applicable where the conduct of research is inherently unsafe/unethical or in a situation in which life is endangered.

- Article 3 (prohibition of torture) – It could be argued that some forms of research are inhuman and degrading. Experimental surgical or drug treatments, with undesirable and/or painful side-effects, might be examples.
- Article 8 (right to respect for private and family life) – Here, challenges could be brought on the basis of informational privacy in relation to research. Also, it might be argued that some observational studies violate the right to privacy.
- Article 10 (freedom of expression) – This could have relevance to those who wish to express concerns about research irregularities or about fraud or the violation of rights in the process of research.
- Article 14 (prohibition of discrimination) – Although there is no right to participate in research, it might be argued that depriving individuals of the benefit of participating in trials, on the basis of their group membership, violates Article 14 on the basis of Article 2, for example. It might also be claimed that some vulnerable groups are over-researched and subjected to unnecessary intrusion, in which case Article 14 might be related to Article 3.

Rights, research and consent

Case 7a

> Alison is a research nurse, working within a medical research team engaged in a drug trial. The trial has two arms – conventional drug and new drug. Alison has been instructed to give patients information about the trial and to recruit as many as possible. One patient/potential research subject asks for further information about treatment options offered and alternatives. Alison responds to some of these questions but is unable to respond to others. The patient also questions the neutrality of the medical team regarding treatment and expresses fears that if he does not agree to participate his care/treatment might be in jeopardy.

This example focuses upon the question of the provision of information. As noted in Chapter 3 above this can be seen as part of respect for the autonomy of the individual patient and bound up with Article 3 of the ECHR. The principle of consent, as discussed in Chapter 2, is generally justified on the basis of respect for autonomy. This can be seen reflected in Article 8 (right to respect for private and family life) and also in relation to other human rights provisions such as Article 3 (prohibition of torture – the right not to be subjected to torture or to inhuman or degrading treatment or punishment). Whilst there is no explicit right to information in relation to research, the professional practice standard has moved towards fuller and franker disclosure of information. There is a movement towards greater provision of information in practice and in research. Further, lack of information might be said to violate Article 8, especially if there is a variation in the information given to different groups.

The BMA (1993 p.208) commented upon the role of nurses in information-giving and consent in research as follows:

'It is often suggested that the patient's consent should be witnessed or that a person other than the researcher should seek patient consent in order to ensure that no pressure is brought to bear. It is generally envisaged that this role be undertaken by nurses but it is sometimes argued that this simply extends the chain of implicit pressure so that nurses feel obliged to cajole patients on behalf of the doctor. The BMA rejects this argument and sees the independence of nurses as a valuable asset in ensuring that pressure is avoided. It is inappropriate for anyone, including a nurse, to be asked to approach patients about consent unless that person has been trained to do so.'

The European Convention on Human Rights contains no specific provisions directed to consent to treatment. Those rights contained in the Convention have thus to be read by implication. In contrast the Council of Europe Convention on Human Rights and Biomedicine, although not binding, makes interesting statements on the question of consent in the context of clinical research (Plomer 2001). Not only does it confirm the importance of informed consent, but it also states in Article 16 that:

'the necessary consent as provided for under Art 5 has been given expressly, specifically and is documented (Article 16 (iii)).'

The issue of consent arises in two places in the trial process; first, in relation to the approval of the clinical trial by the research ethics committee and second, in the context of the operational process of the clinical trial. The REC, in considering the trial protocol, should examine the following issues:

'9.17 Informed consent process

a. a full description of the process for obtaining informed consent, including the identification of those responsible for obtaining consent, the time-frame in which it will occur, and the process for ensuring consent has not been withdrawn

b. the adequacy, completeness and understandability of written and oral information to be given to the research participants, and, when appropriate, their legally acceptable representatives

c. clear justification for the intention to include in the research individuals who cannot consent, and a full account of the arrangements for obtaining consent or authorisation for the participation of such individuals

d. assurances that research participants will receive information that becomes available during the course of the research relevant to their participation (including their rights, safety and well-being)

e. the provisions made for receiving and responding to queries and complaints from research participants or their representatives during the course of a research project.'

In English law, some information must be provided to patients regarding the nature of clinical procedures but, as noted in Chapter 3, there is no general doctrine of informed consent. There is the possibility in relation to some non-therapeutic clinical research procedures that failure to provide full and adequate information may give rise to liability in battery (McHale 1993). In a well-known Canadian case *Haluska v University of Saskatchewan* (1965) 53 DLR 436, the court held that for consent to be valid for the purposes of battery it would be necessary to provide a 'full and frank' disclosure of the facts.

Nonetheless the courts have confirmed that they are increasingly willing to scrutinise the provision of information to patients. While the House of Lords in Sidaway (*Sidaway v Board of Governors of the Bethlem Hospital and the Maudsley Hospital* [1985] 1 AC 871) supported a test for disclosure rooted in that of the responsible body of professional practice, recently judicial statements have been indicative of a different approach. In this case, as we noted in Chapter 3, Lord Woolf commented in *Pearce v Bristol NHS Trust* [1999] PIQR P53 (CA) that:

'If there is a significant risk which would affect the judgement of a reasonable patient then in the normal course it is the responsibility of a doctor to inform the patient of that significant risk, if the information is needed so that the patient can determine for him or herself as to what course that she should adopt.'

It is likely that the courts would be prepared to take certainly no less rigorous approach in the context of the level of disclosure required in therapeutic research.

Moreover, the professional practice standard has moved towards franker and fuller disclosure of information. This is can partly be seen as a natural step in the gradual evolution towards greater provision of information in clinical practice to participants in clinical procedures. However, it can also be seen as something more responsive to particular events. Notable here is the Griffiths Inquiry into a trial of continuous negative extra-thoracic pressure (CNEP) on infants born prematurely at North Staffordshire Hospital during the 1990s (Griffiths 2001). This trial raised concerns regarding the information given to parents involved in the trial and the Inquiry was highly critical of the consent procedures which were adopted.

The emphasis placed upon the importance of information provision by the Griffiths Inquiry is also echoed in the approach of Kennedy in the Bristol Inquiry Report (Kennedy 2001; see further Chapter 3 above). Today it is increasingly difficult for health care professionals to justify withholding information in the context of clinical research. It is now also important to apply the Clinical Trials Directive in this context. This provides for 'informed consent' (Article 3 para 2(b)). It is defined in the Directive as being a decision which is 'taken freely after being duly informed of its nature, significance, implications and risks'. Compliance with the Directive requires that consent must be written, dated and signed. The Directive also addresses the procedural aspects of the consent process requiring that there must be a formal interview undertaken with the investigating team. The aim of the interview is to ensure that participants understand objectives, risks and inconveniences of the trial and their right to withdraw from the trial process. As noted above, while this Directive applies only to medicinal products, in practice its impact is likely to be far broader (Montgomery 2001).

In Case 7a, above, the subject asks questions. While in the context of consent to treatment there is judicial authority to the effect that full responses do not have to be given to questions (*Blyth v Bloomsbury AHA* [1993] 4 Med LR 151) (this has been questioned in later cases e.g. *Pearce v United Bristol Hospitals NHS Trust* [1999] PIQR P53 CA) it is doubtful if that response would ever be legally justified in the context of the research subject asking questions in relation to a clinical trial. The Bristol Inquiry Report (Kennedy 2001) emphasised the need for health care professionals to be responsive to patients' questions. The health care professional would be unwise not to respond fully and frankly to such questions. But what if Alison does not know the answers? It would be suggested as good practice in that situation, first, to admit to the research subject that she does not know the information. Second, she should take steps to ascertain that information and ask other members of the research team.

Alison is told that she must recruit as many people as possible to the trial. This raises the possibility that potential research subjects may be placed under pressure to participate. It is a fundamental principle of English law that consent must be free and unforced (*Re T* [1992] 3 WLR 782). Evidence that consent has been obtained under pressure will invalidate the legitimacy of that consent. Certainly there should be no attempt to discriminate against patients simply because they were unwilling to co-operate in a clinical trial.

The trial in the case study does not include a placebo arm but, if it did, then additional guidelines would apply. The Helsinki Declaration raised implicitly the legitimacy of placebos. The 1996 version of the Declaration provided that all participants in clinical research should 'be assured the best proven diagnostic and therapeutic method'. There was debate regarding this provision as to whether, for example, 'best proven' related to that best proven anywhere in the world or in that particular area. While this has now been changed to 'best current methods...' the meaning of this provision still remains unclear. Forster, Emanuel and Grady (2001) suggest that the current provision does seem to suggest that participants in research studies are entitled to all treatments available in the world, regardless of national priorities, and comment that:

'This is an example of globalisation that could conflict with fair allocation of resources in a country, ultimately making results of research less relevant or useful in certain countries.'

In any event, as we have noted in the resource chapter, the courts have never been prepared to recognise an unlimited right to access health care resources.

A right to protection in research or/and an obligation to intervene?

Case 7b

> *Chris is a registered nurse and research fellow currently engaged in a research project which explores advocacy in a learning disability care setting. The study utilises a variety of methodologies including non-participant observation. In the course of this research, Chris observes a nurse roughly handling a client who has severe learning disabilities.*

The first issue which arises, in this case study, is the legitimacy of this research. It concerns persons with learning disabilities. We noted above the importance of obtaining consent to participation in clinical research in relation to respect for Article 3 and Article 8. But difficulties arise in situations in which the individual lacks capacity to consent.

There are question marks over the legality of the conduct of research on mentally incompetent adults where this are not undertaken for therapeutic purposes. There are also questions about the legality of such procedures. As we noted in Chapter 3, while the House of Lords in *Re F* [1990] 2 AC 1 in 1990 confirmed that clinical procedures may be undertaken upon mentally incompetent adults on the basis of necessity, because it is in their best interests, the application of this judgment to non-therapeutic procedures has been doubted (McHale 1993).

The Law Commission in their 1995 report, 'Mental Incapacity' (Law Commission 1995) recommended the development of a special committee to look at issues concerning the involvement of those with mental incapacity in clinical trials. Their proposals (which were subsequently rejected by the government) however excluded observational studies. But can/should they be excluded from such consideration?

Scrutiny of studies such as the one above by the Research Ethics Committee should ensure that they comply with local, national and international ethical and legal guidelines.

It is also arguable that the integrity of the researcher/nurse is crucial in ensuring that patients'/clients' rights are not violated in the course of such research. There are also now question marks over the legality of the conduct of clinical trials on mentally incompetent adults in the light of the statements made in the Clinical Trials Directive, although this concerns trials on medicinal products. This provides that incompetent adults should only be included where it is essential to undertake research on mentally incompetent adults and the research concerns a life threatening/debilitating condition from which the potential research subject is suffering (Article 5). The Council of Europe, in their Convention on Human Rights and Biomedicine, while it sanctions non-therapeutic research on mentally incompetent adults, contrasts research which may produce results which can confer real and direct benefit on the participants in Article 17(1)(ii) with research 'with the aim of contributing, through significant improvement in the scientific understanding of the individual's condition, disease or disorder to the ultimate attainment of results capable of conferring benefit to the person concerned or to other persons in the same age category or afflicted with the same disease or disorder or having the same condition.' (Article 17(2)(i))

For this type of research to be undertaken it is the case that it entails 'only minimal risk and burden for the individual concerned' (Article 17(2)(ii)). (This Convention while of interest is not presently binding upon the English courts.)

The second issue concerns what Chris should do regarding what appears to be malpractice by the nurse. There is an argument that if Chris does intervene, then this will affect the validity of this particular study. There is no general legal duty to act as a good Samaritan in such a situation. Chris doesn't have direct clinical responsibility for the patients, but he does have obligations as a nurse/researcher. It is clear that the requirements of his roles as researcher and registered nurse may not be compatible. Obviously, he needs to be clear about the nature of what he has observed.

As researcher, Chris endeavours to collect data as a neutral observer without altering what is observed, although this is particularly challenging (see Swanwick 1994; Endacott 1994). However, researchers also have to adhere to codes and declarations designed to protect research subjects from abuse.

The new Research Governance Framework states that:

'Researchers bear the day-to day responsibility for the conduct of research. They are responsible for ensuring that any research they undertake follows the agreed protocol, for helping care professionals to ensure that participants receive appropriate care while involved in research, for protecting the integrity and confidentiality of clinical records and data generated by the research and for reporting any failures in these respects, adverse drug reactions and other events or suspected misconduct through the appropriate systems.' (Para 3.5.1)

In research such as the above it is important to consider, at the design and planning stage of the research project, the possibility of the occurrence of a situation like the one in which Chris finds himself. It would seem prudent to include guidelines about the appropriate response to such a situation within the research protocol.

As a registered nurse, Chris is bound by the NMC Code of Professional Conduct (2002) which states:

'8.2 You must act quickly to protect patients and clients from risk if you have good reason to believe that you or a colleague... may not be fit to practice for reasons of conduct, health or competence...

8.3 Where you cannot remedy circumstances in the environment of care that could jeopardise standards of practice, you must report them to a senior person with sufficient authority to manage them...'

UKCC (1996) guidelines, outlined above, also point out that 'patients should not be exposed to unacceptable risks'. It may be argued that Chris should, in this type of situation, 'blow the whistle' and indeed that this would be part of his professional obligations should internal mechanisms fail. There may also be potential liability depending on the nature of his contract of employment with a university and/or NHS employer.

So is there a right to protection in research and/or an obligation to intervene? The HRA 1998 does not make this right explicit. However, Article 3 could be said to have a bearing on this situation if it is concluded that patients/clients are being subjected to 'degrading or inhuman treatment'. Article 8 might have relevance if it could be argued that the observation violated the patient's/client's right to privacy. The HRA 1998 does not refer to researchers' or professionals' obligations but the NMC Code of Professional Conduct (2002) does.

In addition to urging a consideration of the justifiability of observation as a research method, the case study above also highlights the importance of planning for situations where research subjects are observed to be in jeopardy. Nurses who sit on research ethics committees should be particularly alert to these issues so that the rights of patients/clients can be protected.

'The reality has often fallen short of the ideal.' (BMA 1997 p.220).

Rights, research and the use of human materials

Case 7c

> *Maria is diabetic and expecting her first baby. She is attending the antenatal clinic for a routine check-up. The registrar explains that he is taking blood routinely to check her blood sugar. He also asks Maria if he can take an additional sample for his own research in genetics. Maria agrees without asking further questions.*

This scenario gives rise to the whole question of the legitimacy and retention of human materials for research purposes. This issue has reached public attention with the controversy over the retention of human organs by hospitals leading to the inquiry at Alder Hey Hospital (Report of the Inquiry into the Royal Liverpool Children's Hospital (Alder Hey) (2001) http://www.rclinquiry.org.uk) and the interim inquiry report at Bristol Royal Infirmary (Bristol Inquiry Interim Report Removal and Retention of Human Material (2000) http://www.bristol-inquiry.org.uk). There was widespread storage, not only of organs but, as the census of Professor Liam Donaldson revealed, also of other human material. It is also the case that in addition to tissue from deceased donors, spare human material drawn from living donors may be sought by researchers.

Retention of such material without the consent of the individual (or, in the case of the deceased donor, consent given prior to his death) may constitute an infringement of that person's human rights under Article 8 of the ECHR. Furthermore, such retention and use may also infringe Article 9 in that it constitutes an infringement of the individual's freedom of faith, conscience and of belief. It may furthermore be argued in some situations that retention and use of human materials for purposes which have not been consented for constitutes a violation of Article 3 of the ECHR.

One important issue is the extent to which an individual can ever give up control absolutely over the use of human material, and to what extent generic consent can be regarded as being valid. This issue is a particularly pertinent one at the present time in the light of the establishment of large databases containing genetic information. What form should consent take here? The Human Genetics Commission in their document 'Inside Information' supports the use of generic consent for genetic material where anonymisation has taken place (HGC 2002 para 5.19). The application of a principle of generic consent, whether in relation to tissue or to DNA, is controversial. General consent may be questioned. Maria may consent because that she thinks that the use of her blood for research purposes is to help other patients. However, her view of the situation may change considerably if the registrar intends to use it for a project which leads to considerable commercial gain. Studies have also indicated that patients may have considerable objections to use of their human material without their consent on religious/cultural grounds (Wellcome/MRC 2002).

If the material has not been acquired legitimately then there is the possibility that a patient may subsequently bring legal proceedings. Such an action was brought in the United States in *Moore v University of California* (1990) 793 P2d 479 Cal, by a patient who had had a cell line developed from the use of his spleen without being informed as to this use. While he failed in establishing a property right in that case, he did succeed in establishing absence of informed consent. Nonetheless while in theory such an action may be brought in the UK, in practice such an action may be highly problematic (Dworkin & Kennedy 1993).

The whole question of the regulation of the use of human material is currently the subject of consideration by the Government in a consultation document, 'Human Bodies, Human Choices' (Department of Health 2002). Interestingly, however, this document while mentioning use of tissue for research largely excludes the use of genetic material. Although the regulation of genetic information was considered in the Human Genetics Commission report Inside Information (HGC 2002) it is submitted that there needs to be greater interface between the legal regulation of these areas. It is to be hoped that legislation is introduced to clarify this situation.

Rights, research and children

Case 7d

> *Megan is a paediatric nurse, undertaking a postgraduate nursing degree,*
> *who is required to carry out empirical research in her area of practice. She*
> *is particularly concerned about pain assessment and responses to the pain of*
> *young children following surgery. She is in the process of designing her*
> *research project and, in addition to interviewing and observing staff in*
> *practice, she is considering asking for the views of the children on the ward.*

The involvement of children in research more broadly, or in clinical research, is fraught with controversy. Should children ever be included in research or clinical trials? If so, on what basis? What risks are acceptable? Here Article 3 is of relevance as also is Article 8. In the case above, Megan is considering interviewing young children about their views of pain relief. Is this justifiable? Is there another way to obtain information about pain relief? Could such questioning distress children already distressed by surgery and a strange environment?

The Declaration of Helsinki now also provides in Provision 24 that legally incompetent, incapable persons under the age of majority should not be included in clinical research unless this is necessary to promote the health of the group and is not otherwise attainable with legally competent people. The EU Directive relating to trials on medicinal products enables research to be undertaken on children under tight limits only where:

> 'some direct benefit for the group of patients is obtained from the clinical trial and only where such research is essential to validate data obtained in clinical trials on persons able to give informed consent or by other research methods: additionally such research should either relate to a clinical condition from which the minor concerned suffers or be of such a nature that it can only be carried out on minors.' (Article 4)

While this, as noted earlier, relates to medicinal products, this statement may be influential in relation to the rest of the clinical trials process. Guidance as to the conduct of clinical trials on children has been given by the Royal College of Paediatricians and Child Health (BPA 1992). The RCPCH guidelines have provided that it would not be appropriate to subject a child to a risk which was more than minimal. In relation to trials on medicinal products, the Clinical Trials Directive provides that the design of the trial must be such that it minimises the discomfort, fear and other risks which are foreseeable.

Megan will also be concerned with the issue as to the extent to which the children are to be involved in the consent process. Whose rights are applicable here – the rights of parents or the rights of the child? As we noted in the consent chapter these rights may come into conflict.

As noted in the consent chapter, children over the age of 16 have a statutory right to consent to surgical, medical or dental treatment. Those under 16 may have capacity to consent where they have sufficient maturity to do so (*Gillick v West Norfolk and Wisbech AHA* [1985] 3 All ER 402 HL). It is uncertain, however, to what extent these principles are applicable in relation to clinical trials. The Guidance of the Royal College of Paediatricians and Child Health placed emphasis upon the need for the child's agreement to be obtained. Again, the Clinical Trials Directive is likely to be highly influential outside the area of medicinal products in informing development of the law in this area. In relation to trials on medicinal products the Clinical Trials Directive also provides that information should be given to the child in relation to the child's ability to understand. Also the Directive provides that parents' informed consent should be obtained. It also provides that in a situation in which a child, who has formed a capable opinion, does not want to take part further in the trial then this refusal should not be overridden unless the person conducting the trial has given further consideration to this issue. In English law at present in the context of therapeutic clinical procedures the refusal of a child, of whatever age, can be overridden (*Re R* [1991] 4 All ER 177 and *Re W* [1992] 4 All ER 627). This issue is discussed further above. The extent to which these legal principles represent a conflict between a child's right not to be subject to torture or inhuman and degrading treatment under Article 3, or the right to autonomy under Article 8, remain to be determined. In the case of Megan's project she will need to ensure that appropriate consents are obtained and in practice in such a situation this should surely involve consent of both the child and the parent.

Conclusion

Research is an area infused with the rhetoric of rights, but where the reality of the application of those rights principles is inherently problematic. Much is related to the inherent uncertainties of clinical practice. The NMC (2002) makes reference to research in relation to research-based practice but does not refer explicitly to the role of nurses in research. It may, of course, be argued that guidelines to respect individuality, obtain consent and confidentiality and so on are as applicable to research as a part of professional practice. This is particularly so when nurses are researchers in practice. Given the past atrocities and rights violations in the name of research and continued potential for abuse, there is good reason to be familiar with ethical, legal and professional guidelines regulating this area. The potential of scientific research is enormous. Equally, scientific advances give rise to acute ethical and legal dilemmas. It is still the case that English law in this area is unclear. A human rights framework which strives to preserve life, and to respect human dignity and autonomy surely has a significant role to play in ensuring good research practice.

References

BMA 1993 Medical ethics today – its practice and philosophy. BMJ Publishing Group, London

BMA 2001 The medical profession & human rights – handbook for a changing agenda. Zed Books in association with the BMA, London

Bowling A 1997 Research methods in health: investigating health and health services. Open University Press, Buckingham

British Paediatric Association 2002 Guidelines for the conduct of ethical research involving children. BPA, London

Department of Health 2001 Research governance framework for health and social care. HMSO, London

Department of Health 2002 Human bodies, human choices. DoH, London

Dworkin G, Kennedy I 1993. Human tissue rights in the body and its parts. 1 Medical Review 296

Endacott R 1994 Objectivity in observation. Nurse Researcher 2 (2): 30-40

Forster H P, Emanuel E, Grady C 2001 The 2000 revision of the Declaration of Helsinki: a step forward or more confusion? Lancet 358: 1449

Fox M 2002 Clinical research and patients. In: Tingle J, Cribb A (eds) Nursing law and ethics, 2nd edn. Blackwell Scientific, Oxford

Griffiths R 2001 Report of a research framework in North Staffordshire Hospital NHS Trust. NHS Executive West Midlands Regional Office

Human Genome Commission 2002 Inside information. HGC, London

Keiger D, de Pasquale S 2002 Trials and tribulations. John Hopkins magazine http://www.jhu.edu/~jhuang/0202/web/trials.htm

Kenkre J, Foxcroft D R, McMahon A 2001 Research career pathways. Nursing Standard 16 (4): 39-40

Kennedy I et al 2001 The inquiry into the management and care of children receiving complex heart surgery at the Bristol Royal Infirmary. HMSO, London

Law Commission 1995 Mental incapacity. LCR 231

McHale J V 1993 Guidelines for medical research – some ethical and legal problems. Medical Law Review 1: 160

McHale J, Fox 1997 Health care law text and materials. Sweet & Maxwell, London

Montgomery J 2002 Health care law, 2nd edn. Oxford University Press, Oxford

NMC 2002 Code of Professional Conduct. Nursing & Midwifery Council, London

Plomer A 2001 Medical research, consent and the European Convention on Human Rights and Biomedicine. In: Garwood-Gowers A, Tingle J, Lewis T (eds) Healthcare law: the impact of the Human Rights Act 1998. Cavendish, London

Ramsey S 2000 UK inquiry highlights urgent need for 'research governance'. Lancet 355

Seedhouse D 2000 Practical nursing philosophy: the universal ethical code. John Wiley & Sons, Chichester

Swanwick M 1994 Observation as a research method. Nurse Researcher 2 (2): 4-12

UKCC 1996 Guidelines for professional practice. United Kingdom Central Council for Nursing, Midwifery and Health Visiting, London

Wellcome Trust 2000 Public perceptions of the collection of human biological samples. http://www.wellcome.ac.uk/en/1/biovenpopcol.html

Chapter 8

Rights and the end of life

Introduction

'Diane Pretty loses case, while Miss B "dies with dignity".' (Vertaik 2002)

This headline referred to two high profile end of life cases which appealed to rights in the courts since the incorporation of the HRA 1998 into British law. 42-year-old Diane Pretty, who suffered from motor neurone disease, wanted to take her own life with her husband's help. Mrs Pretty was confined to a wheelchair and was paralysed from the neck downwards. She sought a declaration that her husband should not be prosecuted if he helped her to die. Despite resort to Articles 2, 3, 8, 9 and 14 of the ECHR 1998, her appeal to the House of Lords failed.

Mrs Pretty then took her case to the European Court of Human Rights but she was again unsuccessful. The Court declared that the right to life did not include the right to die. Mrs Pretty subsequently died from her condition on May 11th 2002.

In March 2002, Miss B, a 43-year-old former social care professional, who was quadriplegic, fought a legal battle for the right to have her ventilator turned off (*Re B (adult: refusal of medical treatment)* [2002] 2 All ER 449). This is a notable case although not ultimately decided on the basis of human rights arguments. Doctors at the hospital said that this would be against their ethics. It was ruled that she was mentally competent and had a right to refuse treatment. She died in April 2002 after she was taken off the ventilator.

The NMC Code of Professional Conduct (2002) makes no explicit reference to rights at the end of life but a number of clauses have particular relevance:

'1.3 You are personally accountable for your practice. This means that you are answerable for your actions and omissions, regardless of advice or directions from another professional'

'2.1 You must recognise and respect the role of patients and clients as partners in their care and the contribution they can make to it. This involves identifying their preferences regarding care and respecting these within the limits of professional practice, existing legislation, resources and the goals of the therapeutic relationship'

'2.5 You must report to a relevant person or authority, at the earliest possible time, any conscientious objection that may be relevant to your professional practice. Your must continue to provide care to the best of your ability until alternative arrangements are implemented'; and

'3.2 You must respect patients' and clients' autonomy – their right to decide whether or not to undergo any health care intervention – even where a refusal may result in harm or death to themselves or a foetus, unless a court or law orders to the contrary...'

While respect for patient autonomy is recognised as a key value in the Code, constraints are also highlighted. Respect for autonomy is, for example, curtailed by current legislation. Clause 1.3 outlines the nurse's accountability for actions *and* omissions, which points to the importance of giving as much consideration to non-treatment decisions as to decisions to treat or discontinue treatment. In relation to the commencement, continuation or discontinuation of treatment, there may be situations where the right of nurses to conscientiously object could be applied. In any case, nurses spend a good deal of time with patients and may thus be in a position to come to know what their preferences are regarding treatment and non-treatment and to advocate, where necessary and appropriate, on their behalf.

This chapter will deal with a range of questions relevant to rights and end of life issues. The focus of the chapter is on patients' rights in relation to treatment and non-treatment decision-making, but nurses' rights and the interests of society as a whole may come into issue.

English law makes a distinction between:

- refusing treatment (as in the case of Miss B)
- withholding and withdrawing treatment (as, for example, in the case of Anthony Bland discussed below) – this is sometimes referred to as 'passive euthanasia'
- administering medication intended to end the life of a patient (as in the case of Dr Cox discussed below), described as 'active euthanasia'; and
- requests by a patient that a third party assist in ending their life (as in the case of Mrs Pretty) or 'assisted suicide'.

It is legally permissible for competent adult patients to refuse treatment even if this results in their death. In some situations it is also permissible to withhold and withdraw treatment from the incompetent patient. It continues to be illegal in Britain to intentionally bring about the death of a patient and those who do this are likely to be prosecuted for murder, attempted murder or manslaughter (*R v Cox* [1992] 12 BMR 38). Despite the fact that suicide was decriminalised in Britain by the Suicide Act 1961, assisted suicide remains unlawful under Section 2(1) of the Suicide Act 1961. It seems inevitable that, given the renewed focus on rights brought into being by the HRA 1998, there will continue to be challenges to this situation.

In other parts of the world, there has been a movement towards decriminalising or legalising active euthanasia and assisted suicide in the health care context (Keown 2002). Over a number of years, clinicians in the Netherlands who undertook euthanasia were not prosecuted as long as they followed certain guidelines requiring that:

- the decision was voluntary and well-considered
- the patient was suffering unbearably, and
- a second opinion was obtained.

The operation of these guidelines was not without controversy (Nys 1999). In April 2002, these guidelines were incorporated into legislation explicitly sanctioning euthanasia. The Government in Belgium legalised euthanasia in May 2002. Strict criteria will have to be met before the patient's wish to die can be honoured. The new law gives patients a right to receive ongoing treatment and pain relief, which will be paid for by the State. Further afield, in 1995, the Rights of the Terminally Ill Act, which gave patients a right to seek assistance in dying, became law in Northern Territory, Australia, but was subsequently overturned. In the United States, the Death with Dignity Act 1994 was passed in Oregon, giving patients with six months or less to live the right to ask their doctor for drugs to end their lives. This legislation excluded 'lethal injection, mercy killing and active euthanasia'. It has been reported that the number of terminally ill patients who choose PAS is small: in 1998, there were 16 deaths; in 1999, 27 deaths and in 2000, 26 deaths (Sullivan et al 2001). The effective operation of this legislation in the future has been questioned in the light of Federal legislation which regulates the use of pain-killing drugs. The Federal Attorney General, John Ashcroft, attempted to obtain an injunction so that doctors who assisted suicide would face criminal federal charges. The US Circuit Court overturned the injunction on the grounds that it was unconstitutional. In all of these jurisdictions, whilst doctors are primarily involved in decisions about the administration of life-shortening medication or of withholding or withdrawing treatment, nurses will be closely involved with patients.

Legal challenges regarding rights at the end of life have been and are likely to continue to be brought on the basis of Articles 2 (right to life), 3 (prohibition of torture, freedom from inhuman or degrading treatment), 8 (right to respect for private and family life), 9 (freedom of thought, conscience and religion) and 14 (prohibition of discrimination). So how will the introduction of the rhetoric and practice of rights impact on end of life decision-making in health care?

The right to refuse treatment (adults) – current and advance refusals

Case 8a

> *Sarah is 75 years old and has been admitted to hospital with a recent diagnosis of pancreatic cancer. In discussion with the ward Consultant and her named nurse, she is made aware of the severity of her condition and of treatment options. Sarah says that she does not want any treatment and wishes only to remain pain-free and comfortable. She also tells staff that she has a living will and that, in the event of her losing consciousness, she does not want any life maintenance technologies to be used to revive her. She says: 'I have a right to refuse and to die with dignity.'*

In the case study above, Sarah has been diagnosed as having pancreatic cancer and has been given information about treatment options. Is she competent to make that decision? Although more information is required, it is suggested that Sarah is in a position to understand the implications of her decision, to speak for herself and to refuse treatment verbally. If this is so, then health care professionals are obliged to respect her decisions. The courts in *Re C* [1994] 1 All ER 819 and *Re MB* [1997] 2 FLR 426 and, post-HRA 1998, cases of AK (2002) and *Re B* (adult: refusal of medical treatment) [2002] 2 All ER 449 have confirmed the right of a competent adult to refuse treatment. However, it should also be noted that competence is a decision-relative test: it relates to the gravity of the decision under consideration.

If Sarah is deemed competent, then her treatment refusal should be respected. As indicated above, the Nursing and Midwifery Code (NMC 2002, Section 3.2) highlights the importance of respect for patient autonomy in life and death decision-making. There is a basis for treatment refusal in existing law surrounding battery and consent (*Re T* [1992] 4 All ER 649). Competent individuals have a right to refuse treatment even if this results in their death, although this right is not made explicit in the HRA 1998. A number of recent cases (post-HRA 1998) have reinforced this.

The case of *Re AK (adult patient) (medical treatment: consent)* (Fam Div) 2000 [2001] 2 FLR 35 which involved a 19-year-old male patient who suffered from motor neurone disease highlighted the individual's right to choose. The health trust responsible for his treatment sought a declaration that:

> 'it would be lawful to comply with AK's request to discontinue, two weeks from the date that he lost the ability to communicate, the artificial ventilation and the artificial nutrition and hydration which was being provided to him. AK was able to communicate solely by the movement of one eyelid but this movement would shortly cease. In communicating his wish, by this means, to have the ventilator removed, he had been aware that such action would lead to his death.'

The declaration was granted on the basis that this was a refusal to consent to medical treatment and the patient was an adult of full capacity. It was pointed out that nothing in the Human Rights Act 1998 'vitiated against such a conclusion'.

The case of Miss B, referred to in the introduction, further reinforced the right of competent patients to refuse treatment. In this case, the presiding judge, Dame Elisabeth Butler-Sloss said:

'Unless the gravity of the illness has affected the patient's capacity, a seriously disabled person has the same rights as a fit person to respect for personal autonomy. There is a serious danger, exemplified in this case, of a benevolent paternalism which does not embrace recognition of the personal autonomy of the severely disabled patient.'

A distinction is made in law between those who refuse treatment and those who wish to commit suicide. This was confirmed by the House of Lords in *Airedale NHS Trust v Bland* [1993] AC 789. There has however been some critical comment made of this approach. Keown (2002) has questioned the extent to which refusals which are suicidal can be regarded as being 'different'. He is of the view that 'the right to refuse treatment should be regarded as a shield and not a sword'. We will discuss some of the issues which arise in relation to suicide and assisted suicide in the next section.

It is not always the case that patients/clients are able to express views about health care interventions due to illness and/or incompetence. In the case study, Sarah has anticipated this possibility and has drawn up a 'living will'. This is now more commonly referred to in professional documents as an 'advance statement' ('Making Decisions', LCD 1999).

In an advance statement patients cannot, however, require that professionals do anything illegal (assisted suicide or active euthanasia, for example) nor request that they have treatments which are 'clinically inappropriate'. They can, however, refuse interventions in advance of incompetence. The position of advance refusals is discussed in Section 3.6 of the NMC Code (2002) which states:

'When patients or clients are no longer legally competent and thus have lost the capacity to consent to or refuse treatment and care, you should try to find out whether they have previously indicated preferences in an advance statement. You must respect any refusal of treatment or care given when they were legally competent, provided that the decision is clearly applicable to the present circumstances and that there is not reason to believe that they have changed their minds...'

Advance statements (living wills or advance directives) can be made in a number of ways: by having a discussion with a general practitioner or other health care professional which will be recorded in the patient's notes or more formally, as a written pre-prepared document. Much interest was generated in advance directives with the development of HIV/AIDS. The Terence Higgins Trust produced a standard form living will in conjunction with the

Centre for Medicine Ethics and Law at King's College, London (1991). While the Law Commission in their 1995 report 'Mental Incapacity' did suggest that there should be statutory recognition of advance refusals, this was rejected by the Government in their document 'Making Decisions' (LCD 1999).

Advance statements present challenges for the patient and for professionals caring for the patient. While the law does respect advance refusals, the precise application of advance statements is highly problematic. There is no statutory protection given to advance statements/directives and the existing respect given to them in law comes from common law principles. There are practical challenges also regarding the scope and application of advance statements in an individual context. Health care professionals may, for example, be concerned that following such a statement may lead to the patient's death. There may be uncertainty regarding when the directive was executed and what its scope was. If, for example, an advance statement was made a considerable period of time before the illness/disability developed, would the advance refusal expressed in the directive apply? There may also be anxiety about the patient/client's understanding of the implications of particular illnesses/conditions and their competence at the time of writing. This was commented on in the Royal College of Nursing submission to the Select Committee on Medical Ethics in 1993 (House of Lords, p.83) by Stephen Wright who said:

> 'I think one of our concerns is about the whole nature of these directives. They can only reflect a person's state of mind at the time at which they actually make such a thing, but there is no guarantee or evidence, to show that people who are well and healthy have no problems planning for their death sometimes.'

It is questionable whether individuals can accurately predict what type of treatment they will want in the future. A further issue is what can be refused – does this include palliative care? The Law Commission (1995) supported the approach that a patient should not be able to refuse all 'basic' care. This approach could be considered paternalistic as it negates respect for the autonomy of the individual patient who chooses to forego treatment and care. Interestingly, Section 3.6 of the NMC Code (2002) referred to above states: 'You must respect any refusal of treatment or care'. It is unclear how this will go in the future.

An alternative to an advance statement/directive is the appointment of a proxy decision-maker to assist in clinical treatment decisions. This was supported both by the Law Commission in its 1995 Report (Law Commission 1995) and subsequently by the Government (LCD 1999), although no legislation on this issue has yet been forthcoming. In Scotland, under provisions in the Adults with Incapacity (Scotland) Act 2000, a patient may nominate a proxy decision-maker who will take decisions on their behalf should they become incompetent. As a legal term, 'proxy decision-maker', is not accepted in England and Wales.

In summary then, as a competent adult Sarah has a right to refuse treatment. Should she become incompetent, common law principles support respect for an advance statement of her wishes. Should a rights challenge be necessary in a situation such as this, then it is most likely to be on the basis of Article 8 and possibly Article 3.

Rights and assisted suicide

Case 8b

> *Robert has been receiving palliative care in a medical ward in a general hospital for several months. His partner, Tony, visits every day and tells staff that he would like to take Robert home to die. A nurse overhears a conversation in which Tony promises to get the medication necessary to help Robert to die.*

In cases of assisted suicide, a third party helps an individual to end his/her own life. As stated above, whilst suicide was decriminalised in 1961, Section 2(1) of the Suicide Act 1961 makes it an offence to aid, abet, counsel or procure a suicide. Cases such as that of Diane Pretty have focused discussion on the 'right to die'. Mrs Pretty was diagnosed with motor neurone disease in 1999. She was almost completely paralysed from the neck down but was described as fully mentally competent. Mrs Pretty was unable to take her own life and brought an action to protect her husband from prosecution should he assist her in committing suicide. It was argued that the DPP's refusal to guarantee Mrs Pretty's husband immunity from prosecution should he help her to die, breached her human rights. Mrs Pretty's lawyers contended that Articles 2, 3, 8, 9 and/or 14 of the European Convention on Human Rights required the DPP to give such an undertaking.

At first instance the Divisional Court held that, firstly, the DPP did not have the power to grant an undertaking that he would not prosecute. Secondly, even if he did have that power, any such decision would not be amenable to judicial review. Thirdly, Section 2(1) of the 1961 Act is not incompatible with the ECHR. However, leave was granted to appeal. Three issues were identified by the Divisional Court as being of general public importance. First, does the DPP have power to undertake not to prosecute in advance of the proposed assistance in suicide? Secondly, if he does have that power, taking into account Articles 2, 3, 8, 9 and 14 of the ECHR, was he required not to prosecute Mr Pretty? Thirdly, if not, then was Section 2(1) of the 1961 Act incompatible with Articles 2, 3, 8, 9 and 14 of the ECHR?

In the House of Lords the appeal was dismissed. On the first point it was held that the decision of the DPP not to prosecute was, in exceptional circumstances, amenable to judicial review. But the House of Lords rejected the claims that here Mrs Pretty's rights under the ECHR were being infringed. In relation to Article 2, the principle of the sanctity of life, it was noted in the House of Lords that this was being interpreted very much in terms of a right to self-determination. Lord Bingham commented that:

'If Article 2 does confer a right to self-determination in relation to life and death and if a person were so gravely disabled as to be unable to perform any act whatsoever to cause his or her own death, it would necessarily follow in logic that such a person would have a right to be killed at the hands of a third party without having given help to the third party, and the state would be in breach of the convention if it were to interfere with the exercise of that right. No such right can possibly be derived from an article having the object already defined.'

Furthermore, he stated that:

'Whatever the benefits which, in the view of many, attach to voluntary euthanasia, suicide, physician-assisted suicide and suicide assisted without the intervention of a physician, these are not benefits which derive protection from an Article framed to protect the sanctity of life.'

Moreover it was fundamentally inconsistent with two English law principles the fact that suicide is permissible but that assisted suicide is not.

The House of Lords also held that Article 3, the prohibition on torture and inhuman and degrading treatment, was not applicable. This Article did not impose correlative positive obligations such that the UK was required to ensure that in the case of a competent terminally ill person who wishes but is unable to take their own life that they may seek the assistance of another without being exposed to the risk of prosecution.

In relation to Article 8, this claim was also rejected. Lord Steyn held:

'Counsel submitted that this Article explicitly recognises the principle of the personal autonomy of every individual. He argues that this principle necessarily involves a guarantee as against the state of the right to choose when and how to die. None of the decisions cited in regard to Article 8 assist this argument. It must fail on the ground that the guarantee under Article 8 prohibits interference with the way in which an individual leads his life and it does not relate to the manner in which he wishes to die.'

Lord Bingham also took the approach that the Article applies in relation to:

'protection of personal autonomy while individuals are living their lives and there is nothing to suggest that the article has reference to the choice to live no longer.'

Mrs Pretty held a different view about the weight of autonomy. She said:

'If I am allowed to decide when and how I die, I will feel that I have wrested some autonomy back and kept hold of my dignity...' (Dyer 2002)

The House of Lords also concluded that Article 9 did not entitle Mrs Pretty to manifest her belief in assisted suicide by committing it.

Finally, it was held that Article 14 was not violated because this Article only operated alongside other ECHR rights, and not independently. It was not a general provision against non-discrimination. Lord Steyn also provided an overview of arguments for and against euthanasia and assisted suicide but concluded that 'it is not for us, in this case, to express a view on these arguments'. This very much follows the approach taken by the House of Lords in *Bland* who were of the view that the legitimacy of a law concerning euthanasia was a matter for Parliament and not the courts.

Mrs Pretty took her case to the European Court in Strasbourg but lost this final challenge.

In the European Court of Human Rights, while ultimately here also Mrs Pretty lost, a slightly different approach was taken in relation to Article 8. The ECHR took the view that Article 8 was potentially engaged and that decisions regarding the nature and time of death did fall within the scope of the ECHR.

> 'It is under Article 8 that notions of the quality of life take on significance. In an era of growing medical sophistication combined with longer life expectancies, many people are concerned that they should not be forced to linger on in old age or in states of advanced physical or mental decrepitude which conflict with strongly held ideas of self and personal dignity.'

Nonetheless Article 8 rights are qualified where the limitations are 'necessary in a democratic society', where this is for legitimate reasons and objectives of the legislature and states are accorded a margin of appreciation. In such a situation the need to safeguard the position of the vulnerable in society can justify limitations.

As Article 8 was engaged, consideration could also be given to Article 14, the prohibition on discrimination. Here Article 14 though was not infringed. The discriminatory burden was one which was unavoidable, as otherwise to

> 'seek to build into the law an exemption for those judged to be incapable of committing suicide would seriously undermine the protection of life which the 1961 Act was intended to safeguard and would greatly increase the risk of abuse.'

The judgment in the case of Mrs Pretty led to renewed debate about the legal position of assisted suicide (Keown & Havers in The Times 07/05/02). Keown, for example, referred to a slippery slope argument and argued that the risks of abuse of assisted suicide justified the Court's ruling. Havers, on the other hand, who acted as counsel for Mrs Pretty, argued that the law denied her right to self-determination and that its bid to protect the vulnerable by forbidding assisted suicide disadvantaged a person who is not in need of such protection. He also referred to the distinction made between the cases of Miss B and Mrs Pretty, revisiting the active/passive debate and asked:

> 'Can this distinction really hold? Why is the doctor who switches off Miss B's artificial ventilator in any different position from the person

who places the cyanide pill on Mrs Pretty's tongue? In each case the direct consequence will be death.'

This argument has been supported by academic commentators. Singer (2002) has noted that:

'Technically the lawyers are correct: The two cases cannot be reconciled. They are not inconsistent in the strict meaning of the term. But in a deeper ethical sense the lay observers are right. We have arrived at the absurd situation where a paralysed woman can choose to die when she wants if her condition means that she needs some form of medical treatment to survive, whereas another paralysed woman cannot choose to die when or in the manner she wants because there is no medical treatment keeping her alive in such a way, that, if it were withdrawn she would have a humane and dignified death.'

He also notes that one of the arguments advanced for the distinction is that otherwise pressure would be put upon vulnerable persons were euthanasia to be lawful. However, Singer comments, what of the pressure which could be placed upon vulnerable people to switch off a ventilator? Others however take a different approach.

A further issue is that in our case study. Robert is receiving palliative care but it is not specified if this is adequate. Palliative care developments have done much to improve the quality of care when curative approaches are no longer appropriate. Dame Cicely Saunders is credited with the creation of palliative care when she founded St Christopher's hospice in London in 1967. A definition from the World Health Organisation (1990 cited by Addington-Hall and Higginson 2001 p.240) states:

'[palliative care] is the active total care of patients whose disease is not responsive to curative treatment. Control of pain, of other symptoms, and of psychological, social and spiritual problems is paramount.'

Within this specialty the obligations of professionals are outlined as:

'to relieve pain, symptoms, and suffering; to optimise quality of life; to take into account the uniqueness of individuals, their values, and views and to uphold the dignity of all involved in the dying process.'

A number of national and international rights issues arise in relation to palliative care. It has been pointed out that developing countries have only 5% of the world's total resources for cancer care and yet must deal with almost two thirds of the world's new cancer patients (Faull et al 1998 p.5). The catastrophic effect of AIDS has also highlighted the inadequacy of palliative services. In what is referred to as the 'developed world', it has been argued that there is still

'a major unmet need. The majority of people are not living and dying with the comfort and the dignity that it is possible to achieve for most patients.' (ibid p.6)

Faull et al identify the following specific areas for improvement:

- pain management
- other symptom management
- information and support for patients and carers
- attention to comfort and basic care for those dying in hospital; and
- attention to the needs of patients dying from non-malignant illnesses.

The last point highlights the fact that until recently the focus of palliative care has been on cancer. In cases of motor neurone disease, and perhaps also in the case of Robert above, there appears to be a role for nurses, general and specialist, to assess the need for palliative care and to be instrumental in directing this service to patients in need. It has also been argued that there are deficits in the delivery of palliative care services to those from minority ethnic groups with lower uptake and services which may be 'insensitive and inappropriate to the needs of these groups' (ibid p.6). The difficulty, however, with recognition of health care rights in the context of the Human Rights Act 1998 is that the rights contained in the Act are traditional civil/political rights, not the more recently recognised economic, social and cultural rights. A feature of the latter category is that they frequently involve the expenditure of resources. But traditionally, as was noted in Chapter 7, the courts have been unwilling to intervene to order the expenditure of NHS resources.

Rights and euthanasia

Case 8c

> *Patricia is 45 years old and suffers from breast cancer. She has been told that she now has metastases and she is offered palliative care. Patricia insists that she wishes to die at home and it is agreed that she will have regular visits from the palliative home care team. She has regular doses of diamorphine. She confides in Brenda, one of the nurses, that she wishes to die at a time of her choosing. She asks Brenda if she could give an additional dose of diamorphine 'to finish me off' when the time comes.*

As stated in the introduction, in some parts of the world attempts have been made to decriminalise (active) euthanasia. Whilst euthanasia continues to be illegal in Britain, it is likely that there will be future challenges to the law. There is no explicit reference to a 'right to die' in the ECHR. However, this right has been linked to the right not to be subjected to 'inhuman or degrading treatment or punishment' (Article 3 in HRA 1998) and also to the 'right to respect for private and family life' (Article 8).

Asking someone to 'finish me off' suggests that Patricia is asking for assistance in dying (although as with other case studies, we require more information). A distinction is made between assisted suicide and active euthanasia. As has been pointed out, both are illegal. In the case of assisted suicide, a third party provides the means for an individual to end his/her own life. If Brenda gave Patricia diamorphine tablets, in the knowledge that she wished to use them to end her life, then it might be said that this was an instance of assisted suicide. If, on the other hand, diamorphine was given via a pump and Brenda administered a large dose, as requested, with the intention of ending Patricia's life, it might be said that this was active euthanasia.

In the case of Brenda and Patricia above, the situation is complicated by the administration of medication which is generally intended to alleviate pain. Doctors and nurses are not permitted to help their patients to die but the law allows them to administer pain-killing drugs even though the effect of such administration would be that the patient's life would be shortened. Diamorphine is known to have two effects: on the one hand, it is an effective analgesic when pain is severe and, on the other, it depresses the respiratory centre in the brain, which may shorten life. In *R v Bodkin Adams* [1959] CNM LR 365 Devlin J stated that while patients cannot be 'assisted' to die, pain relief which may shorten life may be allowed:

> 'that does not mean that a doctor who is aiding the sick and the dying has to calculate in minutes or even in hours and perhaps not in days or weeks the effect upon a patient's life of the medicines which he administers or else be in peril of a charge of murder. If the first purpose of medicine, the restoration of health, can no longer be achieved there is still much for a doctor to do and he is entitled to do all that is proper and necessary to relieve pain and suffering even if the measures he takes may incidentally shorten life.'

The doctrine of double effect is cited as justifying this and has been summarised as saying:

> 'on certain conditions, you need not be responsible for those effects of your actions which, though foreseen, are not intended.' (Campbell & Collinson 1988 p.153)

Recently the courts have cast doubt on the principle in this case (*R v Woolin* [1999] 1 AC 82). It remains to be seen if it will be followed in the future in the health care context.

Although the nurse or doctor, then, might foresee that the analgesia may shorten life, the crucial point is that she doesn't intend this outcome. It is the intention of the professional which is said to be crucial in relation to the administration of analgesia and this has received judicial confirmation in later cases (e.g. *Airedale NHS Trust v Bland* [1993] AC 789). The health care professional cannot go that extra mile and administer a dose with the intention of killing the patient.

A further relevant distinction here is between killing and allowing to die. It is held that whilst killing is illegal, allowing a patient to die is sometimes permissible. This is also referred to as active versus passive euthanasia, or as the action versus omission distinction. Legally, professionals may not act to shorten life by, for example, giving a patient a lethal dose of medication, even with benevolent motives (active euthanasia) but may omit (withdraw or withhold) certain treatments or interventions, resulting in the death of the patient/client (passive euthanasia).

These distinctions have been the subject of considerable criticism, not least because they are considered to be hypocritical. In the UKCC submission to the Select Committee on Medical Ethics in 1993, for example, it was argued that:

> 'At the heart of the confusion is the "killing or letting die" distinction. At times this distinction can appear nothing short of hypocritical. Superimposed upon it comes the "intentional killing/alleviating pain" equation. It seems to many nurses, and to this Council, that to prohibit euthanasia as a passive or active measure, yet permit the use of narcotics to alleviate pain, even at doses which will dramatically shorten life or even bring it to a close within a very short period, is no longer a sustainable position.' (House of Lords 1993 p.139)

In *Airedale NHS Trust v Bland* the House of Lords confirmed that the law still recognises the act/omission distinction. Whether Article 8 itself is capable of making a difference here is perhaps questionable. As can be seen in the Pretty judgment, the courts are still holding fast to the sanctity of life principle and its application.

Rights and the withdrawal of treatment from the incompetent patient

Case 8d

> Thomas is 78 years old and suffered severe head and chest injuries in a road traffic accident. He has been unconscious for two months and although he is breathing independently, he requires tube-feeding and is dependent on nursing staff for washing and turning. A diagnosis of permanent vegetative state has been suggested. One of Thomas's sons has said that he would like everything possible done to keep his father alive. Thomas's wife says her husband has a right to die in a dignified manner.

This case raises a number of ethical and legal questions. What rights does someone in PVS have? A right to life? A right to a dignified death? What, if any, rights does the family have? One response is that those in PVS have the same rights as anyone else. Articles in the HRA 1998 begin with 'everyone' and 'no one' and do not say, for example, 'every competent person'. The right to life should not be interpreted as 'everything possible must be done to preserve life regardless'. Rather, it prohibits the intentional taking of life. While the HRA 1998 does not make any explicit reference to a dignified death it may, however, be argued that Article 3, which prohibits inhuman or degrading treatment, supports death with dignity. Article 2 of the HRA 1998 states that 'everyone's life shall be protected by law'. This might lead to the conclusion that everything possible must be done for every patient to safeguard their life regardless of diagnosis, prognosis, professional opinion or individual wishes. Given technological and research developments it is possible that the 'life' of every patient could be maintained indefinitely.

This raises fundamental questions about the value of life and the limits of treatment. The outcome of recent challenges under the HRA 1998, as indicated above, has preserved the status quo, upholding existing law regarding withholding/withdrawing treatment and issues such as euthanasia and assisted suicide.

Before the HRA 1998, the most significant legal ruling in relation to the withdrawal of treatment and sanctity of life was in relation to Hillsborough victim, Anthony Bland (*Airedale NHS Trust v Bland* [1993] AC 789). On the 3rd March 1993 a young Liverpool football supporter, Tony Bland, died of renal failure at Airedale General Hospital in West Yorkshire. He had been in a persistent vegetative state for almost four years as a result of injuries sustained when football fans were crushed against wire fencing at Hillsborough Stadium, Sheffield Wednesday's football ground. In a landmark ruling the House of Lords held that Tony Bland's feeding tube could be withdrawn. The decision was said to have signalled a shift from the traditional sanctity of life view and concluded that tube-feeding could be considered medical treatment which could, in some circumstances, be withdrawn. It was held that Tony Bland should be allowed to die with dignity. The House of Lords discussed the application of the sanctity of life principle now contained in Article 2 of the ECHR.

It has been argued that in this case 'the British courts were breaking with the traditional principle of the sanctity of human life' (Singer 1994 p.73). While a number of cases have confirmed the legal prohibition on active euthanasia, it was recognised that, in some circumstances, it was permissible to withhold treatment where the continuation of that treatment was not in the patient's best interests. The determination of 'best interests' is referable to the Bolam test, namely that of the responsible body of medical practice. The courts have recently taken a broader approach (*Re SL* [2000] 3 WLR 1288) (see further consent chapter above). The support given in the House of Lords for the act/omission distinction is already the subject of heated debate in bioethical literature (see, for example, Rachels 1975, Kuhse & Singer in Harris 2001) and has been referred to in the last section of this chapter. It was argued by Finnis (1993) that their Lordships had indeed crossed the Rubicon in maintaining the distinction between acts and omissions.

Their Lordships' analysis of the sanctity of life principle has been questioned. Keown (1997) suggested that 'sanctity of life was misrepresented, misunderstood and mistakenly rejected' (p.481) and that there was confusion between the terms 'vitalism', 'sanctity of life' and 'quality of life'. Vitalism is the view that 'human life is an absolute moral value and that it is wrong either to shorten it or fail to lengthen it'. Human life must be preserved at all costs. This would have untenable implications for health care and would be likely to violate principles of autonomy, impose burdensome interventions and place an impossible strain on health care resources. Sanctity of life, on the other hand, prohibits killing but it is not an absolute principle. That is, it does not mean that life must be preserved at all costs. Keown suggests that in *Bland* the principle of sanctity of life was confused with vitalism. He suggests that sanctity of life:

> 'offers a middle way between the extremes of vitalism on the one hand and quality of life on the other. Bland represented a swerve towards the quality of life extreme, accepting that certain lives are of no benefit and may lawfully be intentionally terminated by omission.' (p.502)

Keown distinguishes between 'Quality' of life and 'quality' of life. The former he describes as concerned with the 'worthwhileness of the patient's life' whereas the latter he describes as relating to 'an assessment of the patient's condition as a preliminary to assessing the worthwhileness of a proposed treatment'. The former, he argues, 'denies the ineliminable value of each patient and engages in discriminatory judgments, posited on fundamentally arbitrary criteria such as physical or mental disability, about whose lives are "worthwhile" and whose are not'. He suggests that such an approach amounts to discrimination and would seem to violate declarations of human rights. It is arguable that a 'Quality' of life approach does violate Article 14 of the HRA 1998.

Keown suggests that the *Bland* decision also raises the spectre of the slippery slope. He says: 'To the extent that the Law Lords have embraced the quality of life principle, and effectively delegated the judgement on which lives are of no benefit to medical opinion, there is little reason to expect that judgement to be confined to patients in PVS.' He concludes with the recommendation that the withdrawal of treatment and tube-feeding (the care/treatment status of tube-feeding continues to be controversial) from patients in PVS 'should be based on an evaluation of the worthwhileness of the treatment, not the supposed worthwhileness of the patient'.

Here, Keown appears to take quality of life (defined as worthwhileness of the treatment) to be a justifiable part of sanctity of life. Whilst Keown's distinctions and arguments are persuasive, it is not at all clear that an evaluation of the 'worthwhileness of treatment' is a straightforward matter, nor that it can be so clearly distinguished from quality of life, particularly when the patient is incompetent.

The House of Lords held that artificial feeding constituted medical 'treatment' or, as Lord Goff said, 'even if it is not strictly medical treatment, it must form part of the medical care of the patient'. While the case established an important point of principle, allowing the cessation of treatment in such a case, nonetheless their Lordships in *Bland* emphasised that this was an exceptional case and that where subsequent cases arose giving rise to similar difficult ethical issues these should be referred to the Court for determination.

While the House of Lords judgment was controversial, its approach has been followed in other jurisdictions. In a landmark and controversial 1995 ruling in the Republic of Ireland the court sanctioned the withdrawal of nutrition from a woman who had been in a near-persistent vegetative state (*In the Matter of a Ward of Court* [1995] 2 ILRM 401; Feenan 1996). Consideration here was given to constitutional rights including rights to life (an interesting interpretation by Judge Denham encompassing a 'right to die naturally...' p.37) bodily integrity, privacy and self-determination. This case was particularly interesting as it involved a difference of opinion between the family, who sought withdrawal of treatment, and the health care professionals, who opposed withdrawal on the basis of the doctrine of sanctity of life. Nonetheless, the withdrawal of treatment was ultimately sanctioned. This case differed from *Bland* in that the Irish courts did not permit a best interests determination based on what a responsible body of doctors would do. Rather the courts treated the determination of best interests as a question for judicial determination (ibid p.38).

The same principles which are applicable to adults are used in determining cases concerning the withdrawal of treatment from neonates. As indicated in Chapter 2, above, cases which concern children can be some of the most emotive and difficult to determine. The courts have confirmed that treatment may be withdrawn from a child on the grounds that it is in their best interests (*Re J (a minor)(wardship: medical treatment)* [1991] Fam 33). The early cases where treatment withdrawal was confirmed concerned children who were clearly dying (*Re C (a minor)(wardship: medical treatment)* [1981] 1 WLR 1421 CA) – however, in later cases the courts have been prepared to take account of broader guidelines such as those of the Royal College of Paediatricians and Child Health which sanctioned withdrawal not only in a situation in which there was brain stem death or PVS but also where there is 'such severe disease that life-sustaining treatment simply delays death without significant alleviation of suffering or where survival, though possible, would be accompanied by intolerable physical or mental impairment or where, in the face of progressive and irreversible illness, further treatment is more than can be withdrawn' (*Re C (a minor)(medical treatment)* [1998] 1 FLR 1.

Following *Bland* a series of withdrawal of treatment cases have reached the courts and the courts have been prepared to uphold the clinical assessment that treatment should be withdrawn. The almost unquestioning judicial acceptance of clinical judgement in such decisions may lead some to question the effectiveness of the courts as a scrutiniser/determiner of such cases. While in relation to medical negligence and provision of information to patients the courts have indicated that they are more willing to take a critical approach (see consent chapter) there is as yet no evidence of this in relation to end of life decision-making.

Would the enactment of the Human Rights Act make a difference? While their Lordships in *Bland* did consider sanctity of life, the Act was not even a glimmer in the legislator's eye at that time. As far as withdrawal of treatment is concerned, judicial orthodoxy remains. In *NHS Trust A v M* and *NHS*

Trust B v H [2000] 2 FLR 302, Butler Sloss LJ, following the approach taken in *Re A (Children)* [2000] 4 All ER 961 by Robert Walker LJ, ruled that 'intentionally' was a word which should be given its ordinary and natural meaning. She was of the opinion that *Bland* was in accordance with the Human Rights Act 1998 as withdrawal of treatment was an omission, not an intentional deprivation of life. In this case the patient's ultimate death would result from the condition from which she was suffering. Furthermore 'an omission to provide treatment could only violate Article 2 if there was a positive obligation to prolong life, and no such obligation would exist where the patient is in a permanent vegetative state'. Another issue which Butler Sloss LJ considered was the extent to which Article 2 contained a positive obligation to take steps to safeguard life. In this context some consideration was given to the decision in *Osman v UK* (1997) 29 EHRR 245. The Court of Appeal held that the test adopted in this case was analogous to the Bolam test in negligence. In a situation in which a decision was made to withhold treatment because this was not in the patient's best interests, a decision which was supported by a responsible medical opinion, then the state had no further obligation to take adequate steps to safeguard life (Wicks 2001).

Butler Sloss held that Article 3 was inapplicable in relation to those in PVS as it required that the individual was aware of the inhuman or degrading treatment. She also stated that the principles laid down in the *Bland* case were not affected by the Human Rights Act and that as continued artificial feeding was not in the patient's best interests, it could be withdrawn. She was also of the view that Article 8 was inapplicable, as that related to the right to personal autonomy.

The judgment has been criticised by Keown who disputes her interpretation of Article 2, namely that intentional deprivation of life requires an act rather than an omission. He also comments in relation to Article 3:

'Why is it not inhuman or degrading for a doctor to subject an insensate patient to a lingering death from dehydration if the doctor does so to end a life he considers no longer worthwhile?'(ibid p.55)

He also argued that the judgment showed confusion between autonomy and the right to bodily integrity – the latter, he argues, is a right which is possessed by incompetent patients in PVS.

There is one further issue regarding the application of the Human Rights Act and withdrawal of treatment from the incompetent patient which we raise here. The BMA has suggested that it is possible that the present situation, with PVS cases being subject to a court review and other cases not required to, may be inconsistent with the HRA 1998 in relation to discrimination regarding, for example, the right to life (BMA 2001). The BMA states:

'If the courts were to remove the requirement for court review for patients in a persistent vegetative state... this could avoid a potential breach of Article 14. The BMA believe that this is an area that needs urgent review in the light of the Human Rights Act.'

Delaney (2002) also highlights the human rights issues in relation to the review of such decisions to the courts. In *Re C (a baby)* [1996] 2 FLR 43 it was suggested in the High Court that it was not necessary to refer all such cases to the court for determination. However Delaney has suggested that this may infringe the Human Rights Act. She comments that:

> 'our domestic law is now expected emphatically and transparently to protect life. This surely must entail that the decision to let a child die rather than 'inflict' treatment should go to court for an assessment of where the child's best interests lie. Furthermore, explicit criteria will need to be devised to guide decision-making where a child's life is at stake.' (ibid at page 197)

Whilst the Bland case might not have resulted in significant changes in nursing practice, it undoubtedly urged reflection on the meaning of sanctity and quality of life and on the action/omission distinction. Although the ruling emphasised the distinction between actions and omissions (and there continues to be debate as to whether such a distinction can be maintained), it does not follow that nurses are not accountable for their omissions.

The case of Tony Bland raises very fundamental questions about life, death and the purpose of health care. In his case, it was not possible to know for certain how he would have liked to end his life. It needs also to be said that the Bland ruling focused on the situation of patients/clients in PVS and that this was very much a 'one-off case'. However in later cases the courts have been prepared to confirm the decision to withdraw treatment even in situations which depart considerably from the Bland-type situation.

Returning to the example of Thomas with which we opened this section, it is not the case that families have a right to demand either that everything possible is done to keep their loved one alive or to decide that they should be let die. Even in the case of a child, as noted in Chapter 3 above, the parental powers are not unlimited and parents cannot demand the administration of any therapy.

In important respects the case of PVS is more clear-cut. The principles from the Bland ruling require that these cases should be referred for judicial determination. It would also be important to ascertain if Thomas had an advance directive and whether he had expressed a view about his medical treatment in such a situation. Regarding the involvement of Thomas's family in decision-making, there is clearly a disagreement regarding treatment continuation/discontinuation between Thomas's son and his wife. As noted in the consent chapter, the family has no power to consent or refuse on behalf of an adult patient. The treatment is given on the basis of best interests.

Nonetheless that does not mean that in making an assessment of best interests the views of the family will be ignored. Indeed it has been argued that the interests of the family may be a highly relevant consideration in determining what constitutes best interests in any particular situation. In the Bland case, Butler-Sloss LJ said:

> 'The views of the family must always be treated with respect and will be

an important consideration in the overall assessment. In some cases the evidence of relatives will require to be treated with great caution since there may be hidden motives. There is no suggestion that such concerns arise in this family.'

In addition to appreciating the importance of patient autonomy, nurses are also required to 'co-operate with others in the team' (NMC 2002 Section 4). The 'team' includes the patient or client and the patient or client's family. The 2001 BMA guidance also makes reference to the role of family in decision-making. Section 18.3 (p.54) states:

'Even where their views have no legal status in terms of actual decision-making, those close to the patient may have a right to be consulted. In any event it is clear that they can provide important information to help ascertain whether the patient would have considered life-prolonging treatment to be beneficial.'

In fact there is no legal right, at present, for the relatives to be consulted although some may regard it as desirable practice. On the other hand, consulting relatives may in some instances be seen as a violation of confidentiality and an infringement of the privacy of the individual.

The BMA also acknowledge that there may be disagreement amongst relatives, as in the case of Thomas, and that there may exist motives other than the patient's best interests (2001 p.55). The guidance recommends gaining seeking information from more than one person and interpreting it carefully. But in law the views of the relatives are not conclusive and indeed, as in *Re G* [1995] 3 Med LR 80, where there was a disagreement between wife and mother, the courts confirmed clinical judgment in withdrawing treatment.

Conclusion

The rhetoric and the practical application of human rights is considerable in relation to decision making at the end of life. Nonetheless, in this area it may be argued that it may remain as rhetoric still for some considerable time. The cases of Miss B and of AK have further reinforced the patient's right to autonomy. Mrs Pretty's case perhaps illustrates only too clearly the potential of the Human Rights Act 1998, and also its limitations. The movement towards legalising assisted suicide in other European countries suggests that that the last legal word has not been had and that there will continue to be challenges in this most complex and significant area of health care practice. In any case, outside these 'grand' policy and legal decisions the Act itself has much application for nurses seeking to ensure respect the autonomy and dignity of patients in making end of life decisions.

References

Addington-Hall J M, Higginson I J 2001 Palliative care for non-cancer patients. Oxford University Press, Oxford

British Medical Association 2001 Withholding and withdrawing life-prolonging medical treatment – Guidance for decision-making, 2nd edn. BMJ Books, London

Campbell R, Collinson D 1988 Ending lives. Blackwell, in association with The Open University, Oxford

Delaney L 2002 The critically ill patient. In: Tingle J, Cribb A Nursing law and ethics, 2nd edn. Blackwell Scientific, Oxford

Dyer C 2002 Pretty's legal battle for dignity in death. The Guardian 13/05/02 p.9

Faull C, Carter Y, Woof R 1998 Handbook of palliative care. Blackwell Science, Oxford

Feenan D 1996 A 'terrible beauty', the Irish Supreme Court, and dying. European Journal of Health Law 3: 29-48

Finnis J M 1993 Bland crossing the Rubicon. 109 LQR 319

House of Lords 1993-4 Select Committee on Medical Ethics Volume II – Oral Evidence HMSO, London

Keown J 1997 Restoring moral and intellectual shape to the law after Bland. The Law Quarterly Review 113: 481-503

Keown J 2001 Dehydration and human rights. Cambridge Law Journal 53

Keown J 2002a The case of Miss B: Suicide's slippery slope. Journal of Medical Ethics 28: 238

Keown J 2002b Euthanasia: ethics and public policy – an argument against legislation. Cambridge University Press, Cambridge

Keown J, Havers P 2002 Two views on the Diane Pretty case. The Times 7/05.02 p.6

Kuhse H, Singer P 2001 In:Harris (ed) Bioethics. Oxford University Press, Oxford

Law Commission 1995 Mental Incapacity

Lord Chancellor's Department 1999 Making decisions. LCD, London

Nursing and Midwifery Council 2002 Code of professional conduct. NMC, London

Nys H 1999 Physician involvement in a patient's death: A continental European perspective. Medical Law Review 7: 208

Rachels J 1975 Active and passive euthanasia. In: Rachels J (ed) Moral Problems, 3rd edn. Harper Collins, New York

Singer P 1995 Rethinking life and death – The collapse of our traditional ethics. Oxford University Press, Oxford

Singer P 2002 Miss B and Diane Pretty: A commentary. Journal of Medical Ethics 28: 234

Sullivan et al 2001 New England Journal of Medicine 344 (8): 605

Vertaik R 2002 Her message was clear: 'The law has taken all my rights away'. The Independent 30/04/02

Wicks E 2001 The right to refuse medical treatment under the European Convention on Human Rights. Medical Law Review 9: 17-40

Appendix

HUMAN RIGHTS ACT 1998
1998 CHAPTER 42

Long Title

An Act to give further effect to rights and freedoms guaranteed under the European Convention on Human Rights; to make provision with respect to holders of certain judicial offices who become judges of the European Court of Human Rights; and for connected purposes.

Royal Assent [9 November 1998]
Human Rights Act 1998, Ch. 42, Enactment Clause (Eng.)

Enactment Clause 1 The Convention Rights

BE IT ENACTED by the Queen's most Excellent Majesty, by and with the advice and consent of the Lords Spiritual and Temporal, and Commons, in this present Parliament assembled, and by the authority of the same, as follows:—

1 Introduction
    (1) In this Act "the Convention rights" means the rights and fundamental freedoms set out in—
      (a) Articles 2 to 12 and 14 of the Convention,
      (b) Articles 1 to 3 of the First Protocol, and
      (c) Articles 1 and 2 of the Sixth Protocol,
  as read with Articles 16 to 18 of the Convention.
    (2) Those Articles are to have effect for the purposes of this Act subject to any designated derogation or reservation (as to which see sections 14 and 15).

(3) The Articles are set out in Schedule 1.
(4) The [Lord Chancellor] may by order make such amendments to this Act as he considers appropriate to reflect the effect, in relation to the United Kingdom, of a protocol.
(5) In subsection (4) "protocol" means a protocol to the Convention—
(a) which the United Kingdom has ratified; or
(b) which the United Kingdom has signed with a view to ratification.
(6) No amendment may be made by an order under subsection (4) so as to come into force before the protocol concerned is in force in relation to the United Kingdom.

Amendment
Sub-s (4): words "Lord Chancellor" in square brackets substituted by SI 2001/3500, art 8, Sch 2, Pt I, para 7(a).
Date in force: 26 November 2001: see SI 2001/3500, art 1(2).

2 Interpretation of Convention rights

(1) A court or tribunal determining a question which has arisen in connection with a Convention right must take into account any—
(a) judgment, decision, declaration or advisory opinion of the European Court of Human Rights,
(b) opinion of the Commission given in a report adopted under Article 31 of the Convention,
(c) decision of the Commission in connection with Article 26 or 27(2) of the Convention, or
(d) decision of the Committee of Ministers taken under Article 46 of the Convention,
whenever made or given, so far as, in the opinion of the court or tribunal, it is relevant to the proceedings in which that question has arisen.
(2) Evidence of any judgment, decision, declaration or opinion of which account may have to be taken under this section is to be given in proceedings before any court or tribunal in such manner as may be provided by rules.
(3) In this section "rules" means rules of court or, in the case of proceedings before a tribunal, rules made for the purposes of this section—
(a) by the Lord Chancellor or the Secretary of State, in relation to any proceedings outside Scotland;
(b) by the Secretary of State, in relation to proceedings in Scotland; or
(c) by a Northern Ireland department, in relation to proceedings before a tribunal in Northern Ireland—
(i) which deals with transferred matters; and
(ii) for which no rules made under paragraph (a) are in force.

3 Interpretation of legislation

(1) So far as it is possible to do so, primary legislation and subordinate legislation must be read and given effect in a way which is compatible with the Convention rights.

(2) This section—

(a) applies to primary legislation and subordinate legislation whenever enacted;

(b) does not affect the validity, continuing operation or enforcement of any incompatible primary legislation; and

(c) does not affect the validity, continuing operation or enforcement of any incompatible subordinate legislation if (disregarding any possibility of revocation) primary legislation prevents removal of the incompatibility.

4 Declaration of incompatibility

(1) Subsection (2) applies in any proceedings in which a court determines whether a provision of primary legislation is compatible with a Convention right.

(2) If the court is satisfied that the provision is incompatible with a Convention right, it may make a declaration of that incompatibility.

(3) Subsection (4) applies in any proceedings in which a court determines whether a provision of subordinate legislation, made in the exercise of a power conferred by primary legislation, is compatible with a Convention right.

(4) If the court is satisfied—

(a) that the provision is incompatible with a Convention right, and

(b) that (disregarding any possibility of revocation) the primary legislation concerned prevents removal of the incompatibility,

it may make a declaration of that incompatibility.

(5) In this section "court" means—

(a) the House of Lords;

(b) the Judicial Committee of the Privy Council;

(c) the Courts-Martial Appeal Court;

(d) in Scotland, the High Court of Justiciary sitting otherwise than as a trial court or the Court of Session;

(e) in England and Wales or Northern Ireland, the High Court or the Court of Appeal.

(6) A declaration under this section ("a declaration of incompatibility")—

(a) does not affect the validity, continuing operation or enforcement of the provision in respect of which it is given; and

(b) is not binding on the parties to the proceedings in which it is made.

5 Right of Crown to intervene

(1) Where a court is considering whether to make a declaration of incompatibility, the Crown is entitled to notice in accordance with rules of court.

(2) In any case to which subsection (1) applies—
(a) a Minister of the Crown (or a person nominated by him),
(b) a member of the Scottish Executive,
(c) a Northern Ireland Minister,
(d) a Northern Ireland department,
is entitled, on giving notice in accordance with rules of court, to be joined as a party to the proceedings.

(3) Notice under subsection (2) may be given at any time during the proceedings.

(4) A person who has been made a party to criminal proceedings (other than in Scotland) as the result of a notice under subsection (2) may, with leave, appeal to the House of Lords against any declaration of incompatibility made in the proceedings.

(5) In subsection (4)—
"criminal proceedings" includes all proceedings before the Courts-Martial Appeal Court; and
"leave" means leave granted by the court making the declaration of incompatibility or by the House of Lords.

6 Acts of public authorities

(1) It is unlawful for a public authority to act in a way which is incompatible with a Convention right.

(2) Subsection (1) does not apply to an act if—
(a) as the result of one or more provisions of primary legislation, the authority could not have acted differently; or
(b) in the case of one or more provisions of, or made under, primary legislation which cannot be read or given effect in a way which is compatible with the Convention rights, the authority was acting so as to give effect to or enforce those provisions.

(3) In this section "public authority" includes—
(a) a court or tribunal, and
(b) any person certain of whose functions are functions of a public nature,
but does not include either House of Parliament or a person exercising functions in connection with proceedings in Parliament.

(4) In subsection (3) "Parliament" does not include the House of Lords in its judicial capacity.

(5) In relation to a particular act, a person is not a public authority by virtue only of subsection (3)(b) if the nature of the act is private.

(6) "An act" includes a failure to act but does not include a failure to—
    (a) introduce in, or lay before, Parliament a proposal for legislation; or
    (b) make any primary legislation or remedial order.

7 Proceedings

(1) A person who claims that a public authority has acted (or proposes to act) in a way which is made unlawful by section 6(1) may—
    (a) bring proceedings against the authority under this Act in the appropriate court or tribunal, or
    (b) rely on the Convention right or rights concerned in any legal proceedings,
    but only if he is (or would be) a victim of the unlawful act.

(2) In subsection (1)(a) "appropriate court or tribunal" means such court or tribunal as may be determined in accordance with rules; and proceedings against an authority include a counterclaim or similar proceeding.

(3) If the proceedings are brought on an application for judicial review, the applicant is to be taken to have a sufficient interest in relation to the unlawful act only if he is, or would be, a victim of that act.

(4) If the proceedings are made by way of a petition for judicial review in Scotland, the applicant shall be taken to have title and interest to sue in relation to the unlawful act only if he is, or would be, a victim of that act.

(5) Proceedings under subsection (1)(a) must be brought before the end of—
    (a) the period of one year beginning with the date on which the act complained of took place; or
    (b) such longer period as the court or tribunal considers equitable having regard to all the circumstances,
    but that is subject to any rule imposing a stricter time limit in relation to the procedure in question.

(6) In subsection (1)(b) "legal proceedings" includes—
    (a) proceedings brought by or at the instigation of a public authority; and
    (b) an appeal against the decision of a court or tribunal.

(7) For the purposes of this section, a person is a victim of an unlawful act only if he would be a victim for the purposes of Article 34 of the Convention if proceedings were brought in the European Court of Human Rights in respect of that act.

(8) Nothing in this Act creates a criminal offence.

(9) In this section "rules" means—
    (a) in relation to proceedings before a court or tribunal outside Scotland, rules made by the Lord Chancellor or the Secretary of

State for the purposes of this section or rules of court,

(b) in relation to proceedings before a court or tribunal in Scotland, rules made by the Secretary of State for those purposes,

(c) in relation to proceedings before a tribunal in Northern Ireland—

   (i) which deals with transferred matters; and

   (ii) for which no rules made under paragraph (a) are in force,

rules made by a Northern Ireland department for those purposes, and includes provision made by order under section 1 of the Courts and Legal Services Act 1990.

(10) In making rules, regard must be had to section 9.

(11) The Minister who has power to make rules in relation to a particular tribunal may, to the extent he considers it necessary to ensure that the tribunal can provide an appropriate remedy in relation to an act (or proposed act) of a public authority which is (or would be) unlawful as a result of section 6(1), by order add to—

(a) the relief or remedies which the tribunal may grant; or

(b) the grounds on which it may grant any of them.

(12) An order made under subsection (11) may contain such incidental, supplemental, consequential or transitional provision as the Minister making it considers appropriate.

(13) "The Minister" includes the Northern Ireland department concerned.

8 Judicial remedies

(1) In relation to any act (or proposed act) of a public authority which the court finds is (or would be) unlawful, it may grant such relief or remedy, or make such order, within its powers as it considers just and appropriate.

(2) But damages may be awarded only by a court which has power to award damages, or to order the payment of compensation, in civil proceedings.

(3) No award of damages is to be made unless, taking account of all the circumstances of the case, including—

(a) any other relief or remedy granted, or order made, in relation to the act in question (by that or any other court), and

(b) the consequences of any decision (of that or any other court) in respect of that act,

the court is satisfied that the award is necessary to afford just satisfaction to the person in whose favour it is made.

(4) In determining—

(a) whether to award damages, or

(b) the amount of an award,

the court must take into account the principles applied by the
European Court of Human Rights in relation to the award of
compensation under Article 41 of the Convention.

(5) A public authority against which damages are awarded is to be
treated—

(a) in Scotland, for the purposes of section 3 of the Law Reform
(Miscellaneous Provisions) (Scotland) Act 1940 as if the award were
made in an action of damages in which the authority has been found
liable in respect of loss or damage to the person to whom the award
is made;

(b) for the purposes of the Civil Liability (Contribution) Act 1978 as
liable in respect of damage suffered by the person to whom the
award is made.

(6) In this section—

"court" includes a tribunal;

"damages" means damages for an unlawful act of a public authority;
and

"unlawful" means unlawful under section 6(1).

9 Judicial acts

(1) Proceedings under section 7(1)(a) in respect of a judicial act may be
brought only—

(a) by exercising a right of appeal;

(b) on an application (in Scotland a petition) for judicial review; or

(c) in such other forum as may be prescribed by rules.

(2) That does not affect any rule of law which prevents a court from
being the subject of judicial review.

(3) In proceedings under this Act in respect of a judicial act done in
good faith, damages may not be awarded otherwise than to
compensate a person to the extent required by Article 5(5) of the
Convention.

(4) An award of damages permitted by subsection (3) is to be made
against the Crown; but no award may be made unless the appropriate
person, if not a party to the proceedings, is joined.

(5) In this section—

"appropriate person" means the Minister responsible for the court
concerned, or a person or government department nominated by him;

"court" includes a tribunal;

"judge" includes a member of a tribunal, a justice of the peace [(or,
in Northern Ireland, a lay magistrate)] and a clerk or other officer
entitled to exercise the jurisdiction of a court;

"judicial act" means a judicial act of a court and includes an act done
on the instructions, or on behalf, of a judge; and

"rules" has the same meaning as in section 7(9).

10 Power to take remedial action

(1) This section applies if—

(a) a provision of legislation has been declared under section 4 to be incompatible with a Convention right and, if an appeal lies—

(i) all persons who may appeal have stated in writing that they do not intend to do so;

(ii) the time for bringing an appeal has expired and no appeal has been brought within that time; or

(iii) an appeal brought within that time has been determined or abandoned; or

(b) it appears to a Minister of the Crown or Her Majesty in Council that, having regard to a finding of the European Court of Human Rights made after the coming into force of this section in proceedings against the United Kingdom, a provision of legislation is incompatible with an obligation of the United Kingdom arising from the Convention.

(2) If a Minister of the Crown considers that there are compelling reasons for proceeding under this section, he may by order make such amendments to the legislation as he considers necessary to remove the incompatibility.

(3) If, in the case of subordinate legislation, a Minister of the Crown considers—

(a) that it is necessary to amend the primary legislation under which the subordinate legislation in question was made, in order to enable the incompatibility to be removed, and

(b) that there are compelling reasons for proceeding under this section,

he may by order make such amendments to the primary legislation as he considers necessary.

(4) This section also applies where the provision in question is in subordinate legislation and has been quashed, or declared invalid, by reason of incompatibility with a Convention right and the Minister proposes to proceed under paragraph 2(b) of Schedule 2.

(5) If the legislation is an Order in Council, the power conferred by subsection (2) or (3) is exercisable by Her Majesty in Council.

(6) In this section "legislation" does not include a Measure of the Church Assembly or of the General Synod of the Church of England.

(7) Schedule 2 makes further provision about remedial orders.

11 Safeguard for existing human rights

A person's reliance on a Convention right does not restrict—

(a) any other right or freedom conferred on him by or under any law having effect in any part of the United Kingdom; or

(b) his right to make any claim or bring any proceedings which he could make or bring apart from sections 7 to 9.

12 Freedom of expression

(1) This section applies if a court is considering whether to grant any relief which, if granted, might affect the exercise of the Convention right to freedom of expression.

(2) If the person against whom the application for relief is made ("the respondent") is neither present nor represented, no such relief is to be granted unless the court is satisfied—
(a) that the applicant has taken all practicable steps to notify the respondent; or
(b) that there are compelling reasons why the respondent should not be notified.

(3) No such relief is to be granted so as to restrain publication before trial unless the court is satisfied that the applicant is likely to establish that publication should not be allowed.

(4) The court must have particular regard to the importance of the Convention right to freedom of expression and, where the proceedings relate to material which the respondent claims, or which appears to the court, to be journalistic, literary or artistic material (or to conduct connected with such material), to—
(a) the extent to which—
(i) the material has, or is about to, become available to the public; or
(ii) it is, or would be, in the public interest for the material to be published;
(b) any relevant privacy code.

(5) In this section—
"court" includes a tribunal; and
"relief" includes any remedy or order (other than in criminal proceedings).

13 Freedom of thought, conscience and religion

(1) If a court's determination of any question arising under this Act might affect the exercise by a religious organisation (itself or its members collectively) of the Convention right to freedom of thought, conscience and religion, it must have particular regard to the importance of that right.

(2) In this section "court" includes a tribunal.

14 Derogations

(1) In this Act "designated derogation" means—

. . .

any derogation by the United Kingdom from an Article of the Convention, or of any protocol to the Convention, which is designated for the purposes of this Act in an order made by the [Lord Chancellor].

(2) . . .

(3) If a designated derogation is amended or replaced it ceases to be a designated derogation.

(4) But subsection (3) does not prevent the [Lord Chancellor] from exercising his power under subsection (1). . . to make a fresh designation order in respect of the Article concerned.

(5) The [Lord Chancellor] must by order make such amendments to Schedule 3 as he considers appropriate to reflect—

(a) any designation order; or

(b) the effect of subsection (3).

(6) A designation order may be made in anticipation of the making by the United Kingdom of a proposed derogation.

NOTES: Amendment
Sub-s (1): words omitted repealed by SI 2001/1216, art 2(a).
Sub-s (1): words "Lord Chancellor" in square brackets substituted by SI 2001/3500, art 8, Sch 2, Pt I, para 7(b).
Date in force: 26 November 2001: see SI 2001/3500, art 1(2).
Sub-s (2): repealed by SI 2001/1216, art 2(b).
Sub-s (4): words "Lord Chancellor" in square brackets substituted by SI 2001/3500, art 8, Sch 2, Pt I, para 7(b).
Sub-s (4): reference omitted repealed by SI 2001/1216, art 2(c).
Date in force: 1 April 2001: see SI 2001/1216, art 1.
Sub-s (5): words "Lord Chancellor" in square brackets substituted by SI 2001/3500, art 8, Sch 2, Pt I, para 7(b).

15 Reservations

(1) In this Act "designated reservation" means—

(a) the United Kingdom's reservation to Article 2 of the First Protocol to the Convention; and

(b) any other reservation by the United Kingdom to an Article of the Convention, or of any protocol to the Convention, which is designated for the purposes of this Act in an order made by the [Lord Chancellor].

(2) The text of the reservation referred to in subsection (1)(a) is set out in Part II of Schedule 3.

(3) If a designated reservation is withdrawn wholly or in part it ceases to be a designated reservation.

(4) But subsection (3) does not prevent the [Lord Chancellor] from exercising his power under subsection (1)(b) to make a fresh designation order in respect of the Article concerned.

(5) The [Lord Chancellor] must by order make such amendments to this Act as he considers appropriate to reflect—

(a) any designation order; or

(b) the effect of subsection (3).

Amendment

Sub-s (1): in para (b) words "Lord Chancellor" in square brackets substituted by SI 2001/3500, art 8, Sch 2, Pt I, para 7(c).

Date in force: 26 November 2001: see SI 2001/3500, art 1(2).

Sub-s (4): words "Lord Chancellor" in square brackets substituted by SI 2001/3500, art 8, Sch 2, Pt I, para 7(c).

Date in force: 26 November 2001: see SI 2001/3500, art 1(2).

Sub-s (5): words "Lord Chancellor" in square brackets substituted by SI 2001/3500, art 8, Sch 2, Pt I, para 7(c).

Date in force: 26 November 2001: see SI 2001/3500, art 1(2).

16 Period for which designated derogations have effect

(1) If it has not already been withdrawn by the United Kingdom, a designated derogation ceases to have effect for the purposes of this Act—

. . .

at the end of the period of five years beginning with the date on which the order designating it was made.

(2) At any time before the period—

(a) fixed by subsection (1). . ., or

(b) extended by an order under this subsection,

comes to an end, the [Lord Chancellor] may by order extend it by a further period of five years.

(3) An order under section 14(1). . . ceases to have effect at the end of the period for consideration, unless a resolution has been passed by each House approving the order.

(4) Subsection (3) does not affect—

(a) anything done in reliance on the order; or

(b) the power to make a fresh order under section 14(1). . ..

(5) In subsection (3) "period for consideration" means the period of forty days beginning with the day on which the order was made.

(6) In calculating the period for consideration, no account is to be taken of any time during which—

(a) Parliament is dissolved or prorogued; or

(b) both Houses are adjourned for more than four days.

(7) If a designated derogation is withdrawn by the United Kingdom, the [Lord Chancellor] must by order make such amendments to this Act as he considers are required to reflect that withdrawal.

Amendment

Sub-s (1): words omitted repealed by SI 2001/1216, art 3(a).

Date in force: 1 April 2001: see SI 2001/1216, art 1.

Sub-s (2): in para (b) words omitted repealed by SI 2001/1216, art 3(b).

Date in force: 1 April 2001: see SI 2001/1216, art 1.

Sub-s (2): words "Lord Chancellor" in square brackets substituted by SI 2001/3500, art 8, Sch 2, Pt I, para 7(d).

Date in force: 26 November 2001: see SI 2001/3500, art 1(2).

Sub-s (3): reference omitted repealed by SI 2001/1216, art 3(c).

Date in force: 1 April 2001: see SI 2001/1216, art 1.

Sub-s (4): in para (b) reference omitted repealed by SI 2001/1216, art 3(d).

Date in force: 1 April 2001: see SI 2001/1216, art 1.

Sub-s (7): words "Lord Chancellor" in square brackets substituted by SI 2001/3500, art 8, Sch 2, Pt I, para 7(d).

Date in force: 26 November 2001: see SI 2001/3500, art 1(2).

17 Periodic review of designated reservations

(1) The appropriate Minister must review the designated reservation referred to in section 15(1)(a)—

(a) before the end of the period of five years beginning with the date on which section 1(2) came into force; and

(b) if that designation is still in force, before the end of the period of five years beginning with the date on which the last report relating to it was laid under subsection (3).

(2) The appropriate Minister must review each of the other designated reservations (if any)—

(a) before the end of the period of five years beginning with the date on which the order designating the reservation first came into force; and

(b) if the designation is still in force, before the end of the period of five years beginning with the date on which the last report relating to it was laid under subsection (3).

(3) The Minister conducting a review under this section must prepare a report on the result of the review and lay a copy of it before each House of Parliament.

18 Appointment to European Court of Human Rights
(1) In this section "judicial office" means the office of—
(a) Lord Justice of Appeal, Justice of the High Court or Circuit judge, in England and Wales;
(b) judge of the Court of Session or sheriff, in Scotland;
(c) Lord Justice of Appeal, judge of the High Court or county court judge, in Northern Ireland.
(2) The holder of a judicial office may become a judge of the European Court of Human Rights ("the Court") without being required to relinquish his office.
(3) But he is not required to perform the duties of his judicial office while he is a judge of the Court.
(4) In respect of any period during which he is a judge of the Court—
(a) a Lord Justice of Appeal or Justice of the High Court is not to count as a judge of the relevant court for the purposes of section 2(1) or 4(1) of the Supreme Court Act 1981 (maximum number of judges) nor as a judge of the Supreme Court for the purposes of section 12(1) to (6) of that Act (salaries etc);
(b) a judge of the Court of Session is not to count as a judge of that court for the purposes of section 1(1) of the Court of Session Act 1988 (maximum number of judges) or of section 9(1)(c) of the Administration of Justice Act 1973 ("the 1973 Act") (salaries etc);
(c) a Lord Justice of Appeal or judge of the High Court in Northern Ireland is not to count as a judge of the relevant court for the purposes of section 2(1) or 3(1) of the Judicature (Northern Ireland) Act 1978 (maximum number of judges) nor as a judge of the Supreme Court of Northern Ireland for the purposes of section 9(1)(d) of the 1973 Act (salaries etc);
(d) a Circuit judge is not to count as such for the purposes of section 18 of the Courts Act 1971 (salaries etc);
(e) a sheriff is not to count as such for the purposes of section 14 of the Sheriff Courts (Scotland) Act 1907 (salaries etc);
(f) a county court judge of Northern Ireland is not to count as such for the purposes of section 106 of the County Courts Act (Northern Ireland) 1959 (salaries etc).
(5) If a sheriff principal is appointed a judge of the Court, section 11(1) of the Sheriff Courts (Scotland) Act 1971 (temporary appointment of sheriff principal) applies, while he holds that appointment, as if his office is vacant.
(6) Schedule 4 makes provision about judicial pensions in relation to the holder of a judicial office who serves as a judge of the Court.
(7) The Lord Chancellor or the Secretary of State may by order make such transitional provision (including, in particular, provision for a temporary increase in the maximum number of judges) as he considers appropriate in relation to any holder of a judicial office who has completed his service as a judge of the Court.

19 Statements of compatibility

(1) A Minister of the Crown in charge of a Bill in either House of Parliament must, before Second Reading of the Bill—
(a) make a statement to the effect that in his view the provisions of the Bill are compatible with the Convention rights ("a statement of compatibility"); or
(b) make a statement to the effect that although he is unable to make a statement of compatibility the government nevertheless wishes the House to proceed with the Bill.
(2) The statement must be in writing and be published in such manner as the Minister making it considers appropriate.

20 Orders etc under this Act

(1) Any power of a Minister of the Crown to make an order under this Act is exercisable by statutory instrument.
(2) The power of the Lord Chancellor or the Secretary of State to make rules (other than rules of court) under section 2(3) or 7(9) is exercisable by statutory instrument.
(3) Any statutory instrument made under section 14, 15 or 16(7) must be laid before Parliament.
(4) No order may be made by the Lord Chancellor or the Secretary of State under section 1(4), 7(11) or 16(2) unless a draft of the order has been laid before, and approved by, each House of Parliament.
(5) Any statutory instrument made under section 18(7) or Schedule 4, or to which subsection (2) applies, shall be subject to annulment in pursuance of a resolution of either House of Parliament.
(6) The power of a Northern Ireland department to make—
(a) rules under section 2(3)(c) or 7(9)(c), or
(b) an order under section 7(11),
is exercisable by statutory rule for the purposes of the Statutory Rules (Northern Ireland) Order 1979.
(7) Any rules made under section 2(3)(c) or 7(9)(c) shall be subject to negative resolution; and section 41(6) of the Interpretation Act (Northern Ireland) 1954 (meaning of "subject to negative resolution") shall apply as if the power to make the rules were conferred by an Act of the Northern Ireland Assembly.
(8) No order may be made by a Northern Ireland department under section 7(11) unless a draft of the order has been laid before, and approved by, the Northern Ireland Assembly.

21 Interpretation, etc

(1) In this Act—

"amend" includes repeal and apply (with or without modifications);

"the appropriate Minister" means the Minister of the Crown having charge of the appropriate authorised government department (within the meaning of the Crown Proceedings Act 1947);

"the Commission" means the European Commission of Human Rights;

"the Convention" means the Convention for the Protection of Human Rights and Fundamental Freedoms, agreed by the Council of Europe at Rome on 4th November 1950 as it has effect for the time being in relation to the United Kingdom;

"declaration of incompatibility" means a declaration under section 4;

"Minister of the Crown" has the same meaning as in the Ministers of the Crown Act 1975;

"Northern Ireland Minister" includes the First Minister and the deputy First Minister in Northern Ireland;

"primary legislation" means any—

(a) public general Act;

(b) local and personal Act;

(c) private Act;

(d) Measure of the Church Assembly;

(e) Measure of the General Synod of the Church of England;

(f) Order in Council—

(i) made in exercise of Her Majesty's Royal Prerogative;

(ii) made under section 38(1)(a) of the Northern Ireland Constitution Act 1973 or the corresponding provision of the Northern Ireland Act 1998; or

(iii) amending an Act of a kind mentioned in paragraph (a), (b) or (c);

and includes an order or other instrument made under primary legislation (otherwise than by the National Assembly for Wales, a member of the Scottish Executive, a Northern Ireland Minister or a Northern Ireland department) to the extent to which it operates to bring one or more provisions of that legislation into force or amends any primary legislation;

"the First Protocol" means the protocol to the Convention agreed at Paris on 20th March 1952;

"the Sixth Protocol" means the protocol to the Convention agreed at Strasbourg on 28th April 1983;

"the Eleventh Protocol" means the protocol to the Convention (restructuring the control machinery established by the Convention) agreed at Strasbourg on 11th May 1994;

"remedial order" means an order under section 10;

"subordinate legislation" means any—

(a) Order in Council other than one—
  (i) made in exercise of Her Majesty's Royal Prerogative;
  (ii) made under section 38(1)(a) of the Northern Ireland Constitution Act 1973 or the corresponding provision of the Northern Ireland Act 1998; or
  (iii) amending an Act of a kind mentioned in the definition of primary legislation;
(b) Act of the Scottish Parliament;
(c) Act of the Parliament of Northern Ireland;
(d) Measure of the Assembly established under section 1 of the Northern Ireland Assembly Act 1973;
(e) Act of the Northern Ireland Assembly;
(f) order, rules, regulations, scheme, warrant, byelaw or other instrument made under primary legislation (except to the extent to which it operates to bring one or more provisions of that legislation into force or amends any primary legislation);
(g) order, rules, regulations, scheme, warrant, byelaw or other instrument made under legislation mentioned in paragraph (b), (c), (d) or (e) or made under an Order in Council applying only to Northern Ireland;
(h) order, rules, regulations, scheme, warrant, byelaw or other instrument made by a member of the Scottish Executive, a Northern Ireland Minister or a Northern Ireland department in exercise of prerogative or other executive functions of Her Majesty which are exercisable by such a person on behalf of Her Majesty;
"transferred matters" has the same meaning as in the Northern Ireland Act 1998; and
"tribunal" means any tribunal in which legal proceedings may be brought.
(2) The references in paragraphs (b) and (c) of section 2(1) to Articles are to Articles of the Convention as they had effect immediately before the coming into force of the Eleventh Protocol.
(3) The reference in paragraph (d) of section 2(1) to Article 46 includes a reference to Articles 32 and 54 of the Convention as they had effect immediately before the coming into force of the Eleventh Protocol.
(4) The references in section 2(1) to a report or decision of the Commission or a decision of the Committee of Ministers include references to a report or decision made as provided by paragraphs 3, 4 and 6 of Article 5 of the Eleventh Protocol (transitional provisions).
(5) Any liability under the Army Act 1955, the Air Force Act 1955 or the Naval Discipline Act 1957 to suffer death for an offence is replaced by a liability to imprisonment for life or any less punishment authorised by those Acts; and those Acts shall accordingly have effect with the necessary modifications.

22 Short title, commencement, application and extent

(1) This Act may be cited as the Human Rights Act 1998.

(2) Sections 18, 20 and 21(5) and this section come into force on the passing of this Act.

(3) The other provisions of this Act come into force on such day as the Secretary of State may by order appoint; and different days may be appointed for different purposes.

(4) Paragraph (b) of subsection (1) of section 7 applies to proceedings brought by or at the instigation of a public authority whenever the act in question took place; but otherwise that subsection does not apply to an act taking place before the coming into force of that section.

(5) This Act binds the Crown.

(6) This Act extends to Northern Ireland.

(7) Section 21(5), so far as it relates to any provision contained in the Army Act 1955, the Air Force Act 1955 or the Naval Discipline Act 1957, extends to any place to which that provision extends.

SCHEDULE 1 THE ARTICLES
PART I THE CONVENTION

RIGHTS AND FREEDOMS
Article 2
Right to life

1
Everyone's right to life shall be protected by law. No one shall be deprived of his life intentionally save in the execution of a sentence of a court following his conviction of a crime for which this penalty is provided by law.

2
Deprivation of life shall not be regarded as inflicted in contravention of this Article when it results from the use of force which is no more than absolutely necessary:

(a) in defence of any person from unlawful violence;

(b) in order to effect a lawful arrest or to prevent the escape of a person lawfully detained;

(c) in action lawfully taken for the purpose of quelling a riot or insurrection.

Article 3
Prohibition of torture
No one shall be subjected to torture or to inhuman or degrading treatment or punishment.

Article 4
Prohibition of slavery and forced labour

1
No one shall be held in slavery or servitude.

2
No one shall be required to perform forced or compulsory labour.

3
For the purpose of this Article the term "forced or compulsory labour" shall not include:
(a) any work required to be done in the ordinary course of detention imposed according to the provisions of Article 5 of this Convention or during conditional release from such detention;
(b) any service of a military character or, in case of conscientious objectors in countries where they are recognised, service exacted instead of compulsory military service;
(c) any service exacted in case of an emergency or calamity threatening the life or well-being of the community;
(d) any work or service which forms part of normal civic obligations.

Article 5
Right to liberty and security

1
Everyone has the right to liberty and security of person. No one shall be deprived of his liberty save in the following cases and in accordance with a procedure prescribed by law:
(a) the lawful detention of a person after conviction by a competent court;
(b) the lawful arrest or detention of a person for non-compliance with the lawful order of a court or in order to secure the fulfilment of any obligation prescribed by law;
(c) the lawful arrest or detention of a person effected for the purpose of bringing him before the competent legal authority on reasonable suspicion of having committed an offence or when it is reasonably considered necessary to prevent his committing an offence or fleeing after having done so;

(d) the detention of a minor by lawful order for the purpose of educational supervision or his lawful detention for the purpose of bringing him before the competent legal authority;

(e) the lawful detention of persons for the prevention of the spreading of infectious diseases, of persons of unsound mind, alcoholics or drug addicts or vagrants;

(f) the lawful arrest or detention of a person to prevent his effecting an unauthorised entry into the country or of a person against whom action is being taken with a view to deportation or extradition.

2
Everyone who is arrested shall be informed promptly, in a language which he understands, of the reasons for his arrest and of any charge against him.

3
Everyone arrested or detained in accordance with the provisions of paragraph 1(c) of this Article shall be brought promptly before a judge or other officer authorised by law to exercise judicial power and shall be entitled to trial within a reasonable time or to release pending trial. Release may be conditioned by guarantees to appear for trial.

4
Everyone who is deprived of his liberty by arrest or detention shall be entitled to take proceedings by which the lawfulness of his detention shall be decided speedily by a court and his release ordered if the detention is not lawful.

5
Everyone who has been the victim of arrest or detention in contravention of the provisions of this Article shall have an enforceable right to compensation.

Article 6
Right to a fair trial

1
In the determination of his civil rights and obligations or of any criminal charge against him, everyone is entitled to a fair and public hearing within a reasonable time by an independent and impartial tribunal established by law. Judgment shall be pronounced publicly but the press and public may be excluded from all or part of the trial in the interest of morals, public order or national security in a democratic society, where the interests of juveniles or the protection of the private life of the parties so require, or to the extent strictly necessary in the opinion of the court in special circumstances where publicity would prejudice the interests of justice.

2

Everyone charged with a criminal offence shall be presumed innocent until proved guilty according to law.

3

Everyone charged with a criminal offence has the following minimum rights:

(a) to be informed promptly, in a language which he understands and in detail, of the nature and cause of the accusation against him;

(b) to have adequate time and facilities for the preparation of his defence;

(c) to defend himself in person or through legal assistance of his own choosing or, if he has not sufficient means to pay for legal assistance, to be given it free when the interests of justice so require;

(d) to examine or have examined witnesses against him and to obtain the attendance and examination of witnesses on his behalf under the same conditions as witnesses against him;

(e) to have the free assistance of an interpreter if he cannot understand or speak the language used in court.

Article 7
No punishment without law

1

No one shall be held guilty of any criminal offence on account of any act or omission which did not constitute a criminal offence under national or international law at the time when it was committed. Nor shall a heavier penalty be imposed than the one that was applicable at the time the criminal offence was committed.

2

This Article shall not prejudice the trial and punishment of any person for any act or omission which, at the time when it was committed, was criminal according to the general principles of law recognised by civilised nations.

Article 8
Right to respect for private and family life

1

Everyone has the right to respect for his private and family life, his home and his correspondence.

2

There shall be no interference by a public authority with the exercise of this

right except such as is in accordance with the law and is necessary in a
democratic society in the interests of national security, public safety or the
economic well-being of the country, for the prevention of disorder or
crime, for the protection of health or morals, or for the protection of the
rights and freedoms of others.

Article 9
Freedom of thought, conscience and religion

1
Everyone has the right to freedom of thought, conscience and religion; this
right includes freedom to change his religion or belief and freedom, either
alone or in community with others and in public or private, to manifest his
religion or belief, in worship, teaching, practice and observance.

2
Freedom to manifest one's religion or beliefs shall be subject only to such
limitations as are prescribed by law and are necessary in a democratic
society in the interests of public safety, for the protection of public order,
health or morals, or for the protection of the rights and freedoms of others.

Article 10
Freedom of expression

1
Everyone has the right to freedom of expression. This right shall include
freedom to hold opinions and to receive and impart information and ideas
without interference by public authority and regardless of frontiers. This
Article shall not prevent States from requiring the licensing of broadcasting,
television or cinema enterprises.

2
The exercise of these freedoms, since it carries with it duties and
responsibilities, may be subject to such formalities, conditions, restrictions
or penalties as are prescribed by law and are necessary in a democratic
society, in the interests of national security, territorial integrity or public
safety, for the prevention of disorder or crime, for the protection of health
or morals, for the protection of the reputation or rights of others, for
preventing the disclosure of information received in confidence, or for
maintaining the authority and impartiality of the judiciary.

Article 11
Freedom of assembly and association

1
Everyone has the right to freedom of peaceful assembly and to freedom of association with others, including the right to form and to join trade unions for the protection of his interests.

2
No restrictions shall be placed on the exercise of these rights other than such as are prescribed by law and are necessary in a democratic society in the interests of national security or public safety, for the prevention of disorder or crime, for the protection of health or morals or for the protection of the rights and freedoms of others. This Article shall not prevent the imposition of lawful restrictions on the exercise of these rights by members of the armed forces, of the police or of the administration of the State.

Article 12
Right to marry

Men and women of marriageable age have the right to marry and to found a family, according to the national laws governing the exercise of this right.

Article 14
Prohibition of discrimination

The enjoyment of the rights and freedoms set forth in this Convention shall be secured without discrimination on any ground such as sex, race, colour, language, religion, political or other opinion, national or social origin, association with a national minority, property, birth or other status.

Article 16
Restrictions on political activity of aliens

Nothing in Articles 10, 11 and 14 shall be regarded as preventing the High Contracting Parties from imposing restrictions on the political activity of aliens.

Article 17
Prohibition of abuse of rights

Nothing in this Convention may be interpreted as implying for any State, group or person any right to engage in any activity or perform any act aimed at the destruction of any of the rights and freedoms set forth herein or at their limitation to a greater extent than is provided for in the Convention.

Article 18
Limitation on use of restrictions on rights

The restrictions permitted under this Convention to the said rights and freedoms shall not be applied for any purpose other than those for which they have been prescribed.

SECTION 1(3)
PART II THE FIRST PROTOCOL

Article 1
Protection of property

Every natural or legal person is entitled to the peaceful enjoyment of his possessions. No one shall be deprived of his possessions except in the public interest and subject to the conditions provided for by law and by the general principles of international law.
The preceding provisions shall not, however, in any way impair the right of a State to enforce such laws as it deems necessary to control the use of property in accordance with the general interest or to secure the payment of taxes or other contributions or penalties.

Article 2
Right to education

No person shall be denied the right to education. In the exercise of any functions which it assumes in relation to education and to teaching, the State shall respect the right of parents to ensure such education and teaching in conformity with their own religious and philosophical convictions.

Article 3
Right to free elections

The High Contracting Parties undertake to hold free elections at reasonable intervals by secret ballot, under conditions which will ensure the free expression of the opinion of the people in the choice of the legislature.

PART III THE SIXTH PROTOCOL

Article 1
Abolition of the death penalty

The death penalty shall be abolished. No one shall be condemned to such penalty or executed.

Article 2
Death penalty in time of war

A State may make provision in its law for the death penalty in respect of acts committed in time of war or of imminent threat of war; such penalty shall be applied only in the instances laid down in the law and in accordance with its provisions. The State shall communicate to the Secretary General of the Council of Europe the relevant provisions of that law.

SCHEDULE 2
REMEDIAL ORDERS

Orders

1
  (1) A remedial order may—
      (a) contain such incidental, supplemental, consequential or transitional provision as the person making it considers appropriate;
      (b) be made so as to have effect from a date earlier than that on which it is made;
      (c) make provision for the delegation of specific functions;
      (d) make different provision for different cases.
  (2) The power conferred by sub-paragraph (1)(a) includes—
      (a) power to amend primary legislation (including primary legislation other than that which contains the incompatible provision); and
      (b) power to amend or revoke subordinate legislation (including subordinate legislation other than that which contains the incompatible provision).
  (3) A remedial order may be made so as to have the same extent as the legislation which it affects.
  (4) No person is to be guilty of an offence solely as a result of the retrospective effect of a remedial order.

Procedure

2

No remedial order may be made unless—

(a) a draft of the order has been approved by a resolution of each House of Parliament made after the end of the period of 60 days beginning with the day on which the draft was laid; or

(b) it is declared in the order that it appears to the person making it that, because of the urgency of the matter, it is necessary to make the order without a draft being so approved.

Orders laid in draft

3

(1) No draft may be laid under paragraph 2(a) unless—

(a) the person proposing to make the order has laid before Parliament a document which contains a draft of the proposed order and the required information; and

(b) the period of 60 days, beginning with the day on which the document required by this sub-paragraph was laid, has ended.

(2) If representations have been made during that period, the draft laid under paragraph 2(a) must be accompanied by a statement containing—

(a) a summary of the representations; and

(b) if, as a result of the representations, the proposed order has been changed, details of the changes.

Urgent cases

4

(1) If a remedial order ("the original order") is made without being approved in draft, the person making it must lay it before Parliament, accompanied by the required information, after it is made.

(2) If representations have been made during the period of 60 days beginning with the day on which the original order was made, the person making it must (after the end of that period) lay before Parliament a statement containing—

(a) a summary of the representations; and

(b) if, as a result of the representations, he considers it appropriate to make changes to the original order, details of the changes.

(3) If sub-paragraph (2)(b) applies, the person making the statement must—

(a) make a further remedial order replacing the original order; and

(b) lay the replacement order before Parliament.

(4) If, at the end of the period of 120 days beginning with the day on which the original order was made, a resolution has not been passed

by each House approving the original or replacement order, the
order ceases to have effect (but without that affecting anything
previously done under either order or the power to make a fresh
remedial order).

Definitions

5
In this Schedule—
"representations" means representations about a remedial order (or
proposed remedial order) made to the person making (or proposing to
make) it and includes any relevant Parliamentary report or resolution; and
"required information" means—
> (a) an explanation of the incompatibility which the order (or proposed
> order) seeks to remove, including particulars of the relevant declaration,
> finding or order; and
> (b) a statement of the reasons for proceeding under section 10 and for
> making an order in those terms.

Calculating periods

6
In calculating any period for the purposes of this Schedule, no account is to
be taken of any time during which—
> (a) Parliament is dissolved or prorogued; or
> (b) both Houses are adjourned for more than four days.

[7
> (1) This paragraph applies in relation to—
>> (a) any remedial order made, and any draft of such an order
>> proposed to be made,—
>>> (i) by the Scottish Ministers; or
>>> (ii) within devolved competence (within the meaning of
>>> the Scotland Act 1998) by Her Majesty in Council; and
>> (b) any document or statement to be laid in connection with such an
>> order (or proposed order).
> (2) This Schedule has effect in relation to any such order (or proposed
> order), document or statement subject to the following
> modifications.
> (3) Any reference to Parliament, each House of Parliament or both
> Houses of Parliament shall be construed as a reference to the
> Scottish Parliament.
> (4) Paragraph 6 does not apply and instead, in calculating any period for
> the purposes of this Schedule, no account is to be taken of any time
> during which the Scottish Parliament is dissolved or is in recess for
> more than four days.]

Amendment
Para 7: inserted by SI 2000/2040, art 2(1), Schedule, Pt I, para 21.
Date in force: 27 July 2000: see SI 2000/2040, art 1(1).

SCHEDULE 3
DEROGATION AND RESERVATION

Part I . . .

. . .

NOTES:
Amendment
Repealed by SI 2001/1216, art 4.
Date in force: 1 April 2001: see SI 2001/1216, art 1.

Sections 14 and 15
Royal Assent [9 November 1998]
Human Rights Act 1998, Ch. 42, Sch. 3, Pt. I (Eng.)

[Part I Derogation]

[United Kingdom's derogation from Article 5(1)
The United Kingdom Permanent Representative to the Council of Europe
presents his compliments to the Secretary General of the Council, and has
the honour to convey the following information in order to ensure
compliance with the obligations of Her Majesty's Government in the
United Kingdom under Article 15(3) of the Convention for the Protection
of Human Rights and Fundamental Freedoms signed at Rome on 4
November 1950.

Public emergency in the United Kingdom
The terrorist attacks in New York, Washington, DC and Pennsylvania on
11th September 2001 resulted in several thousand deaths, including many
British victims and others from 70 different countries. In its resolutions
1368 (2001) and 1373 (2001), the United Nations Security Council
recognised the attacks as a threat to international peace and security.

The threat from international terrorism is a continuing one. In its
resolution 1373 (2001), the Security Council, acting under Chapter VII of
the United Nations Charter, required all States to take measures to prevent
the commission of terrorist attacks, including by denying safe haven to
those who finance, plan, support or commit terrorist attacks.

There exists a terrorist threat to the United Kingdom from persons
suspected of involvement in international terrorism. In particular, there are
foreign nationals present in the United Kingdom who are suspected of

being concerned in the commission, preparation or instigation of acts of international terrorism, of being members of organisations or groups which are so concerned or of having links with members of such organisations or groups, and who are a threat to the national security of the United Kingdom.

As a result, a public emergency, within the meaning of Article 15(1) of the Convention, exists in the United Kingdom.

The Anti-terrorism, Crime and Security Act 2001
As a result of the public emergency, provision is made in the Anti-terrorism, Crime and Security Act 2001, inter alia, for an extended power to arrest and detain a foreign national which will apply where it is intended to remove or deport the person from the United Kingdom but where removal or deportation is not for the time being possible, with the consequence that the detention would be unlawful under existing domestic law powers. The extended power to arrest and detain will apply where the Secretary of State issues a certificate indicating his belief that the person's presence in the United Kingdom is a risk to national security and that he suspects the person of being an international terrorist. That certificate will be subject to an appeal to the Special Immigration Appeals Commission ("SIAC"), established under the Special Immigration Appeals Commission Act 1997, which will have power to cancel it if it considers that the certificate should not have been issued. There will be an appeal on a point of law from a ruling by SIAC. In addition, the certificate will be reviewed by SIAC at regular intervals. SIAC will also be able to grant bail, where appropriate, subject to conditions. It will be open to a detainee to end his detention at any time by agreeing to leave the United Kingdom.

The extended power of arrest and detention in the Anti-terrorism, Crime and Security Act 2001 is a measure which is strictly required by the exigencies of the situation. It is a temporary provision which comes into force for an initial period of 15 months and then expires unless renewed by Parliament. Thereafter, it is subject to annual renewal by Parliament. If, at any time, in the Government's assessment, the public emergency no longer exists or the extended power is no longer strictly required by the exigencies of the situation, then the Secretary of State will, by Order, repeal the provision.

Domestic law powers of detention (other than under the Anti-terrorism, Crime and Security Act 2001)
The Government has powers under the Immigration Act 1971 ("the 1971 Act") to remove or deport persons on the ground that their presence in the United Kingdom is not conducive to the public good on national security grounds. Persons can also be arrested and detained under Schedules 2 and 3 to the 1971 Act pending their removal or deportation. The courts in the United Kingdom have ruled that this power of detention can only be exercised during the period necessary, in all the circumstances of the

particular case, to effect removal and that, if it becomes clear that removal is not going to be possible within a reasonable time, detention will be unlawful (R v Governor of Durham Prison, ex parte Singh [1984] 1All ER 983).

Article 5(1)(f) of the Convention
It is well established that Article 5(1)(f) permits the detention of a person with a view to deportation only in circumstance where "action is being taken with a view to deportation" (Chahal v United Kingdom (1996) 23 EHRR 413 at paragraph 112). In that case the European Court of Human Rights indicated that detention will cease to be permissible under Article 5(1)(f) if deportation proceedings are not prosecuted with due diligence and that it was necessary in such cases to determine whether the duration of the deportation proceedings was excessive (paragraph 113).

In some cases, where the intention remains to remove or deport a person on national security grounds, continued detention may not be consistent with Article 5(1)(f) as interpreted by the Court in the Chahal case. This may be the case, for example, if the person has established that removal to their own country might result in treatment contrary to Article 3 of the Convention. In such circumstances, irrespective of the gravity of the threat to national security posed by the person concerned, it is well established that Article 3 prevents removal or deportation to a place where there is a real risk that the person will suffer treatment contrary to that article. If no alternative destination is immediately available then removal or deportation may not, for the time being, be possible even though the ultimate intention remains to remove or deport the person once satisfactory arrangements can be made. In addition, it may not be possible to prosecute the person for a criminal offence given the strict rules on the admissibility of evidence in the criminal justice system of the United Kingdom and the high standard of proof required.

Derogation under Article 15 of the Convention
The Government has considered whether the exercise of the extended power to detain contained in the Anti-terrorism, Crime and Security Act 2001 may be inconsistent with the obligations under Article 5(1) of the Convention. As indicated above, there may be cases where, notwithstanding a continuing intention to remove or deport a person who is being detained, it is not possible to say that "action is being taken with a view to deportation" within the meaning of Article 5(1)(f) as interpreted by the Court in the Chahal case. To the extent, therefore, that the exercise of the extended power may be inconsistent with the United Kingdom's obligations under Article 5(1), the Government has decided to avail itself of the right of derogation conferred by Article 15(1) of the Convention and will continue to do so until further notice.
Strasbourg, 18 December 2001]

NOTES:

Amendment
Inserted by SI 2001/4032, art 2, Schedule.
Date in force: 20 December 2001: see SI 2001/4032, art 1.

Amendment
Inserted by SI 2001/4032, art 2, Schedule.
Date in force: 20 December 2001: see SI 2001/4032, art 1.

Index